Strategies for Survival

Strategies for Survival

A Gay Men's Health Manual
for the Age of AIDS

by

Martin Delaney and Peter Goldblum
with Joe Brewer

Illustrated by Howard Cruse

St. Martin's Press
New York

Library of Congress Cataloging-in-Publication Data

Delaney, Martin.

    Strategies for survival.
    1. AIDS (Disease)—Prevention. 2. Homosexuals,
Male—Health and hygiene. I. Goldblum, Peter.
II. Title. [DNLM: 1. Acquired Immunodeficiency
Syndrome—prevention—popular works. 2. Homosexuality—
popular works. WD 308 D337s]
RC607.A26D45 1987   616.97'9205   87-4504
ISBN 0-312-00558-X (pbk.)

First Edition

10 9 8 7 6 5 4 3 2 1

Contents

Dedication —

This book has been a way for us to come to grips with our own vulnerability to AIDS and the ways in which it has touched our lives. We dedicate it to our lovers, Kenny and Mark, whose courage and struggles to survive have inspired this work, and to all the men, women, and children who have lived with or taken part in the battle against AIDS.

Peter Goldblum
Martin Delaney

Acknowledgments

Contributing Authors:
Some chapters of this book include essential contributions from subject-matter experts in our community. Without their help, the quality this book would be diminished. Contributions include:

Barbara Faltz, contributor: Substance Use and Abuse
    Former coordinator, AIDS Substance Abuse Program, UCSF AIDS Health Project; Training Coordinator for the School of Nursing, UCSF AIDS Professional Education Project; Author, "Substance Abuse as a Co-factor to AIDS" in *What to Do about Aids: Physicians and Mental Health Professionals Discuss the Issue,* UC Press.

David Doyle, contributor: Exercise
    YMCA Fitness Professional, Associate Director of Health Enhancement and Fitness Trainer; swimming Coach for the International Gay Games I and II.

Lois Borgmann, R.D., MPH., contributor: Nutrition
    Public Health Nutritionist, San Francisco, Dept. of Public Health; nutritional consultant to persons with AIDS and AIDS related agencies.

Les Morgan, contributor: Resources—Appendix
    Co-chair, National Information Systems Task Force, a joint project of the National AIDS Network, the San Francisco AIDS Foundation, and several other major AIDS agencies; Les is also a manager of technology planning for a major pharmaceutical company.

Design and Layout:
Jim Tetzlaff, graphic designer, whose keen sense of design makes this book readable and functional, and who helped craft its diverse parts into a coherent whole.

Other Contributors:
This book, truly a product of the gay community, evolved over several years, beginning as a guide for support group leaders and later evolving into the comprehensive work it is today. So many have given generously of their time and knowledge that it is impossible to credit all of them here. To name a few:
- *Howard Cruse,* our illustrator, whose sensitivity to the material and commitment to our community typifies the involvement which is heralded in this book
- *Dr. Kenneth Payne* for reviews and suggestions which kept us anchored in the real world;
- *Dr. Patrick McGraw* and the late *Dr. David Winterhalter,* for their ongoing reviews;
- *Mark Montgomery,* for his pragmatic critique and word processing of evolving chapters;
- *Michael Denneny,* at St. Martin' Press, for his concern for our community and his gracious patience in allowing this book to come to fruition without the usual demands of deadlines or the attitude of "that's good enough."
- The men and women of the Prevention Section of the UCSF AIDS Health Project, who, by sharing freely of their experience in support groups, contributed to the early stages of development: *John Acevedos, Ernest Andrews, Gary Dexter, Marcia Quackenbush, Tim Sally, William Vitiello,* and *Joseph Wilson;*
- *The San Francisco AIDS Foundation,* for providing seed money to support the early projects which lead to this book.

PREFACE

The AIDS crisis is testing the gay community in ways many of us would not have believed possible only a few short years ago. Virtually every gay man living in a major city now knows someone who is ill or has died. In many cases, people have lost a significant number of friends in a very short period of time. By any standards, this is unnatural. We are faced with the almost unbearable spectacle of people in their twenties and thirties scanning the obituary pages each day for the names of their peers. It is a scenario analogous only to wartime.

Yet in the first terrible years of the epidemic, the people affected most directly by it were left to handle the crisis virtually without the support of government institutions or established social service agencies. If it hadn't been for the early efforts of community-based organizations such as New York's Gay Men's Health Crisis and The San Francisco AIDS Foundation, the existence of AIDS would have been totally ignored until it began to enter the general population.

Even now, much of the world fails to fully comprehend the enormity of what is taking place in the gay community and how difficult it has been for us to cope with such a crisis on a daily basis. It is neither productive nor desirable to set up an "us" and "them" situation. After all, many heterosexuals have been personally touched by AIDS and have become deeply involved, just as many in the gay community have retreated into denial and apathy. We are all in this together. Yet it must be acknowledged that our minority status as gay people brings an added dimension to the problem. Some of the difficulties we face in this crisis are those faced by everyone. Others are particular to gay people and must be dealt with in the context of our history as an oppressed community.

Consider for a moment how our relatives might react if *their* friends, neighbors, and families began dying at such a terrifying rate. Imagine, for example, several nuclear families of your acquaintance being wiped out in less than a few months. Your loved ones would be crazed—living in a daily state of emergency—and you would be expected to understand and share their overwhelming grief. Yet gay families and gay relationships are given so little legitimacy that our suffering is minimized and somehow devalued.

Many lesbians and gay men are frightened, confused, and numb with grief. Worse, too many of them are still spectacularly uninformed, living lives governed by misinformation, rumor, and irrational fear. Yet in a few short years this crisis has also galvanized a fragmented, often politically divided community, and has sparked courage, generosity, and commitment beyond anything we could have foreseen.

This book is designed to help gay people cope with the AIDS crisis by teaching us how to emerge from the darkness of ignorance and fear into the light of knowledge and action. But it is not enough just to cope. It is also necessary for us to wake each other up and finally begin to take our health into our own hands. We must break out of our paralysis and fight not only for our own lives but for the lives of the people we love.

When this nightmare is over—and it *will* be over someday—the gay community will survive. And the generations of gay people who come after us will look back on a group of people who dared much that others might live. The stories of those individual people will be the stories of men and women who were able to heal themselves both emotionally and physically. This book is a battle plan for that healing and for the anger that must follow. Use it.

> *- Vito Russo*

FOREWORD

When the first reports of a strange new disease began spreading through the gay communities of the East and West coasts in 1981, no one had the slightest notion of the frightful human drama which was about to unfold. Each passing year since then has increased both our knowledge of the epidemic and our awareness of its gravity. Despite significant strides made on the medical front, a true cure still remains beyond our grasp and an effective vaccine is, at best, years away. Today, as then, public education and personal responsibility are our most potent weapons. They will remain so for the foreseeable future.

Collectively, educational efforts have already impeded the growth rate of the disease. Yet, the number of new diagnoses is still doubling every year in most cities, every 8 or 9 months in some. Cities which had a small problem in 1983 are now experiencing the near geometric rates of progression seen in New York, San Francisco, and Los Angeles in the early years of the epidemic.

We are now faced with the prospect of increased spread to additional risk groups, most ominously that of urban minority youth. Solid evidence exists of transmission outside of the known risk groups, and the acknowledged means of transmission has been broadened to include heterosexual intercourse.

On the bright side, we are witnessing the first glimmers of hope regarding treatments. There is evidence that life can be prolonged and that progression to the more deadly forms of the disease can be slowed. Yet these are limited victories, affecting only the speed with which AIDS takes its victims.

Even with such progress, even if a vaccine were announced tomorrow instead of five or ten years hence, we would still have a catastrophe ahead of us. It is estimated that as many as two million people are *already* infected—and that number increases daily. The latest research indicates that a large number of those will go on to develop the disease.

Education and personal responsibility are our most potent weapons and we must make the most of them. Simple guidelines are not enough. Instead, each individual needs to know where he or she stands and what to do about it. When the assessment of individual risk is high, a personal plan for survival must be established.

This book, the most comprehensive of its type I have seen, provides a much-needed mechanism for coping. It offers no quick solutions, no facile reassurances. Yet it does provide hope, hope based on knowledge and reason, not denial. It gives individuals a means of understanding and controlling risks, a means of weeding through the growing volumes of often contradictory advice, a way of personally doing something about the epidemic.

The concepts represented here have enormous implications for public health—not just as a response to AIDS, but for the entire spectrum of sexually transmitted diseases. It provides a toolkit for people who are already ill, people who are newly infected, people who are simply scared. The fact that it comes from and builds upon the gay community's experiences in this epidemic is a fitting memorial to the tragic suffering so many have experienced. Let's hope that its message and strategies can help prevent others from sharing in that suffering.

James W. Dilley, M.D.
Project Director, AIDS Health Project,
and Assistant Clinical Professor of Psychiatry,
University of California, San Francisco.

PURPOSES OF THIS BOOK

This book is designed to help gay men accomplish several objectives:

- to better UNDERSTAND WHAT HEALTH IS and how to maintain it;

- to EVALUATE YOUR PERSONAL RISK for contracting AIDS;

- to help you decide WHAT CHANGES, IF ANY, YOU WANT TO MAKE in key aspects of your life which affect your health;

- to LEARN A PLANNING PROCESS for implementing change;

- to better RECOGNIZE THE THREAT OF AIDS to ourselves and our community, and to encourage you to take a stand in facing that threat.

To achieve these objectives, it is necessary to read:

- this introduction, "USING THIS BOOK;"

- the first chapter, "HEALTH IN THE AGE OF AIDS;"

- any or all of the middle chapters which address your own needs and concerns regarding AIDS;

- the final chapter, "FIGHTING FOR OUR LIVES," which addresses issues of great concern to all members of our community.

The first chapter presents the basic definitions, assumptions, and tactics of the book. After reading it, you can read any or all of the chapters which follow, *in any sequence you wish.* Some of the topics may already be well understood by those readers who are most familiar with AIDS and may thus be of lesser interest to them. For others who are coming to grips with these issues for the first time, all chapters may be important. You are encouraged to focus on the subjects which you feel are most important to your personal health. The final chapter, intended for all readers, deals with our community and individual responses to the universal challenges we face in living through the epidemic.

Subject Matter

Chapter 1, "HEALTH IN THE AGE OF AIDS" discusses the meaning of health itself and how our community has been affected by the AIDS crisis. This chapter lays out the basic beliefs upon which this book is based. It also looks at the often conflicting approaches to health we encounter. Three general groups of people are addressed throughout this and subsequent chapters:

• people currently ill with AIDS or ARC;

• people not currently ill with AIDS or ARC but who have tested positive to the AIDS antibody (often called "sero-positives");

• people not ill with AIDS or ARC, who are either antibody negative or untested, yet concerned with the epidemic.

The first chapter also introduces a four-step planning process for establishing a personal health plan, a means of *doing something* about the challenges we face. This health planning model is then applied in each of the key subject areas addressed in subsequent chapters.

The middle chapters address the major lifestyle issues that affect health, including:

SEXUAL PRACTICES–(Chapter 2)

THE ROLE OF STRESS–(Chapter 3)

SUBSTANCE USE AND ABUSE–(Chapter 4)

SOCIAL SUPPORT–(Chapter 5)

EXERCISE AND NUTRITION–(Chapter 6)

The final chapter, "FIGHTING FOR OUR LIVES" (Chapter 7), discusses strategies for meeting the overall threat—medical, political, and psychological—AIDS poses to our community. In support of this theme, an appendix entitled "RESOURCES" is provided to direct readers to the remarkable body of AIDS-related support services, organizations, and references which have evolved in and around the gay community.

The Activity Process   The introductory chapter of this workbook is intended primarily as reading material—a somewhat passive experience. As such, it will only require a small time commitment. Reading it is essential for making good use of this book.

The chapters dealing with specific health behaviors, such as those on "SEXUAL PRACTICES" or "THE ROLE OF STRESS," include both text and learning activities. As you read the text, you will be asked to stop at times to complete practical exercises. These are designed to provide a systematic process for improving your health, one which looks inward for self-assessment and outward for planning change.

The action-planning model is presented in the belief that taking action—not passive reading and intellectual understanding—is required if we are to meet the challenges before us. Many readers will find it helpful to use the action exercises as presented to apply what is learned. Some may prefer to simply do the reading and internalize the concepts in their own way. Broad experience in AIDS/ARC support groups suggests that the action exercises play a critical role in making lasting changes and implementing effective strategies.

Whatever action you decide to take, it will be enacted in the form of commitments—commitments you make to yourself, about yourself, at your own choosing. You will not, however, be asked to give up the pleasures of life. On the contrary, this book encourages you to get on with your life— sexually, psychologically, politically, and spiritually. If we let fear of AIDS drive us back into the closets and abandon the freedoms we've struggled centuries to achieve, we will surrender to the homophobic demands of our enemies. We must find a way to cope with the threat of AIDS without giving up our identities and freedoms. This book is intended as guidebook on that journey.

You may choose to use this workbook alone as a personal and private activity, or you may choose to work with a group of close friends or acquaintances. Much of what is contained here is based on the experiences of gay health workshops and support groups. Working in a group provides several important benefits, including:

• learning from the experiences of others;

• getting and giving support, understanding, and reinforcement;

• meeting new and interesting people who share your concerns and outlook;

• discovering that your fears and anxieties are neither crazy, unique, nor unsolvable.

While the group approach has advantages over individual activity, the book is structured to work either way. The key to success is using the book in an ACTIVE manner, involving yourself in the thought processes, reflection, and personal planning exercises.

Benefits

Use of the exercises and planning processes presented here have been shown to provide many important benefits:

• reduced risk and lowered anxiety regarding AIDS;

• improved sexual, social, and emotional outlook;

• a better balanced perspective from which to evaluate health and healing options;

• greater sense of purpose and a better understanding of our roles as part of a community under seige;

• renewed spirit to live our lives proudly and fully as gay men.

Like just about everything else in life, you'll only get as much out of the book as you put into it. Openness, candor, and caring for yourself and others will help make the time you spend with it well worthwhile.

A Gay Health Perspective

What Is Health?

Healing, Prevention, and Promotion

Approaches to Health

Steps to a Healthier Future

CHAPTER

1

HEALTH IN THE AGE OF AIDS

A GAY HEALTH PERSPECTIVE

Don Clark, in his book *Loving Someone Gay,* has pointed out why many gay people are skeptical of those who tell us that we need to change our behaviors. Many of us have heard the opinions of "experts" who tried to change us in ways that went against our best interests or that we knew just wouldn't work. In many cases, their suggestions were based on anti-gay assumptions. Now, as we face a crisis that forces us to seek both scientific expertise and medical advice, we find that our skepticism creates a dilemma:

Where do we get information we can believe?

Who should we trust?

Who has our best interests at heart?

In the present crisis, we need the best and most up-to-date information available—and a way to evaluate it. It's aggravating to listen to authorities today who don't really understand our culture. We've had to learn to be skeptical, to think critically, to challenge and explore the underlying assumptions of any advice that encourages us to make changes. The intentions and assumptions which underlie this book, even though written by gay people, should be examined by the reader before deciding if the strategies and suggestions are appropriate.

The content of this book is based on the following assumptions:

ASSUMPTION 1:
  Gayness—homosexuality—is a naturally occurring and common form of human behavior.

ASSUMPTION 2:
  Sexual behavior is an important and valuable aspect of the human experience.

ASSUMPTION 3:
  The pressures placed on gay men and lesbians by a hostile society make extra demands on us which can NEGATIVELY affect our health. Conversely, feeling good about ourselves as gay people can POSITIVELY affect our health.

Over the last two decades, our community has experienced tremendous growth and development. We've seen the seeds of a proud and upfront community, sown by the previous generation, grow and flourish. Instead of hiding within society the way we were forced to in the past, we now live our lives openly. We have our own culture, neighborhoods, restaurants, theaters, services, and political representation. Perhaps most importantly, we have a degree of self-respect and personal pride that has been denied us in the past. Of course, there's still room for growth and improvement—there always will be. The benefits of an open society are not equally available in all locations. Gay people in small towns and more conservative cities sometimes face a more hostile environment. Even in our major population centers, "tolerance" is not always the same as unquestioned "acceptance."

Men and women loving, living, and relating openly to members of the same sex is still a fairly new experience. While the practice of homosexuality has been around throughout history, its open acceptance and acknowledgement have not. There is much to learn yet, both on our part and on the part of those who see us as "different."

Most of us still grow up with the negative view of homosexuality taught and reinforced by churches, parents, and government. This must be overcome personally—externally and internally—before we can have a solid, unshakable sense of our self-worth.

Because of the resistance we've faced throughout our lives, courage has become a central aspect of being gay. Each step of our individual and community growth has required the courage to stand alone and make our own way. We are now in the midst of a new chapter of our development, one which brings us new challenges and opportunities. We are regularly being called upon to make choices about what is best for us at a time when there are no absolute or final answers. The goal of this book is to assist us in making these choices and putting them into action.

WHAT IS HEALTH?

Perhaps at no time in history have so many people paid such close attention to health. In the past twenty years, our basic understanding of health has expanded enormously. Health is no longer viewed merely as the absence of disease, but now incorporates our physical, psychological, social and spiritual well-being.

For the purposes of this book, health can be defined at three different levels. At the most basic, most physical level:

LEVEL ONE: *Freedom from disease or injury and any limitations they impose on us.*

At this level, we are healthy if the functions of our organs, including our cells and bones, are not disrupted or impaired. Staying healthy at this level primarily means preventing contact with the agents of disease and avoiding situations which might threaten us physically.

While this level of health is certainly desirable, it doesn't fully reflect our complexity as human beings. Thus a second level of health must be described.

At the second level, the integration of our physical parts is taken into account. Here, health is:

LEVEL TWO: *Our human systems working together, functioning effectively as a unit.*

At this level, it isn't required that each part is functioning as it should. Here, the successful interaction of the elements as a system is the measure of health.

Staying healthy at this level requires attention not only to the physical condition of the parts of our bodies, but also to how they function together as a unit. Second-level health care includes increased attention to exercise, nutrition, stress, and the substances we ingest.

Viewing health from this perspective has many advantages. It allows us to recognize that we are more than the sum of our parts. And, more importantly, it helps us realize that *we can be healthy without being perfect.* Imperfections in any individual parts of the body may be compensated for by other elements of the system. Strength in one area may offset weakness in another. Health at this level means capitalizing on our strengths and assets and adapting to our deficiencies.

The degree of health represented by this second level is vitally important, but it too falls short of addressing the whole being. There is another aspect of our humanity which also plays a major role in health. Thus a third level of health can be described.

At the third, and most uniquely human level, another complex aspect of our being is addressed—our intellect, feelings, actions, and spirituality. At this level, health is:

LEVEL THREE: *An experience, a state of mind in which we are at peace or in harmony with ourselves and our physical and social environment.*

Health extends beyond the body and its physical functioning. Here, our physical, social, and spiritual realities interact to achieve a state of health.

Staying healthy at this level requires attention to both of the previously mentioned levels and to our emotions, attitudes, feelings, and beliefs. Health care must address our psychological needs, our sense of meaning and purpose, our notions of right and wrong (values), and our ability to give and receive love.

It is on this plane of health that we finally get around to viewing health as *concerning the whole being.* As in LEVEL TWO, health here allows us to understand both our strengths and limitations, to recognize what's good about us and what's not. It allows us to accept ourselves and others as we truly are.

One author, Fritjof Capra, defined health as:

"*. . . the experience of well-being resulting from a dynamic balance that involves the physical and psychological aspects of the organism, as well as its interactions with the natural and social environment.*" (*The Turning Point, 1983*)

Other authors might use different words to describe it, but the message is clear:

HEALTH CONCERNS THE WHOLE BEING

This complete picture of health, sometimes known as the "biopsychosocial" model, incorporates each of the key aspects of our humanity:

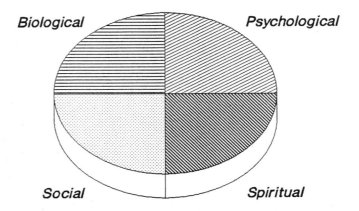

This book subscribes to this all-encompassing view of health.

HEALING, PREVENTION, PROMOTION

To fully understand the view of health which guides this book, it's important to note the distinctions between HEALING, PREVENTION, and PROMOTION.

Healing

When someone is ill, he may be "unhealthy" at any of the three levels discussed. If infection or injury disrupts the body, there is a problem at the first level of health. If the interaction of the human systems fails in some way, there is a problem at the second level of health. If a person lacks a sense of well-being or wholeness, there is a problem at the third level of health. Wherever the problem, something must be done to correct it. This is the process of HEALING—making things better, fixing what's wrong.

Discussions of health in our culture have traditionally focused on healing. Western society has long viewed illness as being caused by germs, fractures, viruses, and genetic or organic disorders. As science has advanced, physicians have learned how to repair many disorders. We have come to expect that all forms of illness sooner or later will yield before medicine's sword.

AIDS, however, has shaken our faith in the science of medicine. Despite years of frantically struggling with the disease in laboratories and hospitals, a true cure has yet to be found or even predicted. The culprit has been named—the HIV virus (previously called HTLV III and LAV)—but still no "magic bullet" has been found to stop it.

Research groups have described the HIV (AIDS virus) infection as causing a spectrum of diseases, not just AIDS. This means that all who have it are infected by the same organism, but can have very different type of resulting illness. Previously, four categories were recognized:

- SEROPOSITIVE (tested positively to HIV virus, but no signs of illness are present)

- LAS (lymphadenopathy syndrome, or swollen lymph nodes but no other symptoms)

- ARC (AIDS-Related Condition, often including LAS but with other infections or symptoms as well, such as oral thrush, etc.)

- AIDS (any of the above plus one of another of a list of problems experienced by AIDS patients, such as pneumocystis pneumonia, Kaposi's Sarcoma—KS—etc.)

Some groups now divide this into six levels of HIV infection, each of which describes a different stage of the disease. Although we don't yet have a complete picture of how the disease works, it is increasingly clear that one stage of the disease often leads to another. In the early years of the epidemic, it was believed that only a small percentage of the people who were infected (seropositive) would eventually go on to develop ARC or AIDS. Likewise, it was believed that only a small percentage of those with ARC would develop full-blown AIDS. Longer-range studies now paint a much grimmer picture of this progression, suggesting that most who are seropositive will develop some degree of illness, and that people with ARC very often progress to AIDS.

Many believe that this frightening picture of a predictably progressive disease only holds true if nothing is done to counteract the illness, either by lifestyle changes or treatment. Recent advances in medicine for the first time make it possible to slow the deterioration experienced by AIDS patients and to slow the progression to AIDS from LAS or ARC (or from lower level HIV infection to higher). Yet people treated with such medicines still have the illness and require constant medication. Thus, we are as yet unable to achieve health on the first level, since the organism is still troubled. Likewise, health on the second level is imperfect because the body systems still aren't interacting as they are intended. Since there is no medical "cure" for the disorder of AIDS, we need to look to the healing possible on the other levels of health.

To achieve healing despite HIV infection requires focusing our attention primarily on the third level of health described above. On this level, healing is possible despite imperfections in our bodies and in our science. We can have health on this level while living with disorders on the lower levels. Such an outlook can maximize our sense of control over the illness, and thus, over our health itself.

Interestingly, health at this level has been shown to boost health at the lower levels. Psychological, emotional, and spiritual health have long been known to have an impact on the solely physical aspects of health. The powers of healing often associated with this third and higher level of health have been profound for many people.

Although we can't fully understand the mechanisms involved in this type of healing, we can choose to leave this door (and our minds) open to it, to let it work for us. Or we can close the door and wait for the "magic bullet." This is a choice we each must make individually.

Degrees of healing can take place on any of the three levels of health. Some may choose to concern ourselves with only one level or another, and that is our right. The people most experienced with healing—AIDS patients themselves—typically encourage us to use whatever we find that helps, to open our minds to new ideas and concepts. Finally, they encourage us to share what we know and what we learn with others in the community who might benefit from our experiences. This too may be part of the power of healing.

Prevention

Another consequence of our failure to find a cure for AIDS is the need to direct our efforts toward PREVENTION. While we have no easy solution to offer those who are already showing later stages of HIV infection, we do know enough about the disease to slow its spread to others. Those actions we take, both individually and as a community, to prevent further spread of the disease, are forms of PREVENTION.

PREVENTION can also work at all three levels of health. There are things we can do at LEVEL ONE to avoid coming into the contact with the agent, the virus, which causes AIDS. There are things we can do to minimize the risk of transmitting it to others. At LEVEL

TWO, we can take action to strengthen our defensive systems against the attack of the virus. At LEVEL THREE, we can examine the role our attitudes, emotions, and beliefs play in resisting disease.

This knowledge, on all levels, brings with it a great responsibility.

For many, the knowledge of what's needed for PREVENTION has posed a severe dilemma. Many of the freedoms and behaviors we fought for under the banner of civil rights are now implicated in the spread of disease. Rabid homophobes seem to view AIDS with special delight, seeing in it a vindication of their fears, a justification for their long-held prejudices. They seem more preoccupied with homosexuality and its practices than homosexuals have ever been.

The challenge for us is twofold:

1. *Acknowledge and respond effectively to what's known about transmission of the disease. . .*

2. *. . . yet do so without abandoning our freedom or accepting the guilt a homophobic society would lay at our feet.*

Promotion

We can take action to prevent further spread of disease. We can attempt healing of the whole being, if not of the disease itself. Finally, we can act in ways which PROMOTE health in the fullest sense.

Health PROMOTION can be described as positive actions to create an environment where health is possible. PROMOTION operates from our understanding of health on the third level. By recognizing our complexity as physical, spiritual, psychological, and social beings, we can create a personal environment which makes HEALING most possible. With careful thought and planning, we can create an environment in which PREVENTION need not mean abandoning our natural desires and fundamental needs.

Norman Cousins, former editor of *The Saturday Review*, describes in his book *Anatomy of an Illness* how he promoted his own health using a collage of methods. While wrestling with a life-threatening illness, he took actions ranging from the chemical to the comical to supplement the recommendations of his doctor. His self-designed therapy included massive injections of Vitamin C, heavy doses of positive mental outlook, and a regimen of laughter induced by re-runs of "The 3 Stooges" movies. He credited his eventual recovery in part to the combined effect of all the actions he took. Although his methods may or may not be meaningful to you, the importance of health promotion is deeply underscored by his experiences.

A healthful environment is one which recognizes our uniqueness as human beings, one which acknowledges our physical, intellectual, social, and emotional nature. Each of us is both an individual and a member of a community. A healthful environment supports our needs for social contact, intimacy, and emotional satisfaction.

Creating a healthful environment means making the most of our connections with:

- our surroundings,

- our lovers, families, and circle of friends,

- the community of gay people everywhere,

- the community of humankind.

Although we don't always recognize it, each of the key elements can make a contribution to our health when they are in balance.

APPROACHES TO HEALTH

If science had been able to quickly find the "magic bullet" cure for AIDS, we might be less concerned with exploring the alternative paths to health. If there were a single, surefire way to cure or prevent this disease, we would all be lining up to take advantage of it.

Because the "magic" hasn't been found, we are instead faced with choosing from a bewildering array of options, none of which comes with a guarantee. The uncertainties we face are so strong that, as a rule of thumb, we can easily distinguish sincerity from quackery:

> —*the quacks are the ones who are sure they can cure us.*

Despite the good intentions of most of those offering help, some people have used the crisis to make personal gains at the expense of the sick and the frightened. As AIDS/ARC patients, or as the "worried well," we can easily be naive to the real intentions of promoters of "remedies." Yet on another level, we can just as easily misjudge people who sincerely offer help when they do so from a view of science, health, or healing which differs from our own.

Those who have heard the numbing diagnosis of AIDS or ARC from their doctors are quickly confronted with a limited range of choices from which to confront the illness. Sometimes it seems as if the sick are asked to choose a position on a mythical spectrum of approaches to health and treatment, ranging from science to mysticism.

THE MYTHICAL SPECTRUM OF HEALING

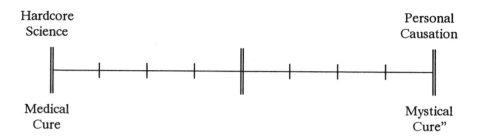

Hardcore Science

Medical Cure

Personal Causation

Mystical Cure"

Practitioners at one end of the scale express grave doubts about those at the other. Each can make believable arguments about why they're right and the others are wrong. Both want to take responsibility for the "cure."

But is this view accurate? Must we really choose between them? Let's examine what each, hypothetically, is saying.

The "Hardcore Science" Approach

At one end of the spectrum lies the purely physical, rationalist views of Western medicine. In this view, which operates primarily on a *level one* understanding of health, disease is caused by a physical agent, the AIDS virus. It must be fought with the tools of physics, chemistry, and biology. At its extreme, this view contends that anything which can't be seen or measured simply doesn't exist, or is irrelevant. The cure for disease is sought in the lab using sophisticated and expensive equipment, following time-honored methods of science. Until a true cure is found, hardcore science would limit participation by the sick or at-risk population to involvement as research subjects in formal experimental protocols. Everyone else must "wait and see."

In this view of medicine, physicians and researchers are the ultimate authorities and lead actors in the drama of healing. Physicians not involved in the search for the cure treat the day-to-day symptoms as they arise with approved medicines. Patients typically take a less active role in their own treatment, doing only what they're told—no questions asked. Any pursuit of unapproved treatments or alternative healing is met with condescension or ridicule.

WHAT'S WORKING RIGHT HERE? There is little doubt that disease is indeed caused by harmful agents such as bacteria and viruses. And, historically, the science of medicine has ultimately been successful in combating thousands of other diseases. Most of us believe, or need or want to believe, that science will eventually find a cure. And progress has indeed been made against AIDS, particularly in the treatment of opportunistic infections.

WHAT'S MISSING IN THIS PICTURE? Unfortunately, hardcore science has had little success in finding an effective protocol for AIDS or ARC. While progress has been made in extending life and slowing progression of the illness, the disease lives on, unconquered. "Hardcore science" provides little assurance to those who wait—other than the hope that, based on previous successes, science will eventually find a cure. It fails to acknowledge several important alternatives:

- the healing powers found on *level three* of health;

- the lessons of Eastern medicine;

- patient access to promising, but not yet approved therapies;

- the value of hope in helping people hold on until a cure is found.

In short, "hardcore science" is reluctant to recognize the value of things which don't fit under its microscope or which it hasn't taken the time to examine.

The "Personal Causation" Approach

At the other extreme of the spectrum are those who reject or downplay the importance of the physical agents of disease. In this view, the patient is asked to take responsibility for his or her illness. Disease is seen as a symptom of spiritual, emotional, or psychological distress. This distress may either be the result of choices the patient has made or the effects of cruel and unfair pressures imposed by an unfriendly environment. From this perspective, hope springs from the ability of the individual to make different choices, to choose a path of wellness instead of a path of sickness. Healing power is said to be in the hands of the individual—not the doctors and scientists.

Surprisingly, the notion of "personal causation" is applied to AIDS by groups of widely differing and often conflicting viewpoints. Some of its most obvious proponents can be found on the "religious right," the peddlers of fundamentalist religious morality. For them, AIDS is their god's punishment for the sin of homosexuality. The "cure," which is most often delivered only in the afterlife, can only come about through repentance and suppression of the patient's homosexual desires. In exceptional cases, if their god allows, the patient just might be allowed to return to health through a "miracle." Such miracles might even be timed for the convenience of the TV viewing audience shortly before the collection plate is passed. Fundamentalist practitioners of "personal causation" have raised perhaps as much money by exploting AIDS as we have in all our benefits and fundraising galas.

But not only the "religious" right adhere to theories of personal causation and mystical cure. Others hold a similar view from a humanistic and sympathetic perspective. For these, the failure is not one of offending a deity, but some vaguely defined natural order. The problem is not necessarily homosexual behavior, but perhaps a poor self-image, harmful nutritional practices, or psychological problems and various forms of self-abuse brought about as a response to living in a hostile, homophobic society. The patient can cure himself by changing the behavior patterns which lead to disease, by better coping with the hostility. While this attitude may be less judgmental, the principles of self-causation and mystical self-healing remain the cornerstone.

WHAT'S WORKING RIGHT HERE? Nothing is right in the "religious right's" vicious attacks. But in a broader sense, this viewpoint recognizes the importance of personal responsibility in the healing process. The "hardcore science" extreme puts responsibility (and thus hope) for healing in the hands of the scientist, leaving the patient a helpless pawn. Practitioners of "personal causation" sometimes can help people regain control of the healing process. Likewise, this approach has more room in it for alternative healing and alternative medicine, thus making it possible for patients to make use of all the resources available to them, not just those sanctified by science.

WHAT'S MISSING IN THIS PICTURE? Unfortunately, this outlook may have the harmful effect of placing blame for illness on the patient. The resulting guilt and remorse may further complicate the illness since they place additional stress and burdens on the patient. Failure to cure the disease is sometimes seen as a personal failure. Religious zealots conveniently ignore the fact that people who are "good," even by their standards, get AIDS, while most people who are "bad" don't. They look the other way when confronted with the fact that lesbians are statistically the least likely of all to be victimized by AIDS—and thus must be God's chosen people. Of course, their god "works in mysterious ways."

Any approach—whether it be "personal causation," holism, or Eastern mysticism—which minimizes the value of the remedies offered by modern medicine is likely to do the patient a dangerous disservice. When a gay man comes down with pneumocystis pneumonia, sending him to a health food store, the confessional, to a mystic healer, or anywhere other than the hospital, is irresponsible.

Choosing a Personal Path — A Balanced Approach

Clearly, there's a wide gap between "hardcore science" and mysticism. Fortunately, many of our physicians and spiritual leaders have been anxious to help us see all the opportunities and possibilities. A practical approach doesn't ask us to choose a position on the spectrum, but rather to choose a path which works for ourselves..

Many of the people who have lived longest with AIDS, or who have successfully resisted its onset, have chosen personal paths which combine insights from the "hardcore science" and "personal causation" approaches, and from the broad area in between. They take the best of conventional and alternative medical approaches, spiritual resources, psychological remedies, and make good use of the social support offered by their loved ones. They avoid letting one loud voice overrule the others. They are driven by their courage rather than their fear, and choose to see the positive aspects of the steps they take without shirking responsibility for their mistakes.

In short, they form a personal, integrated approach which parallels the *bio-psycho-social* model of health described previously.

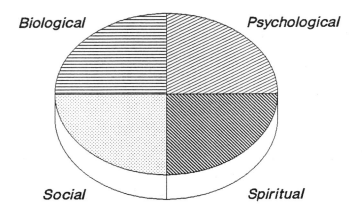

BIOLOGICAL—

Learn about and consider the biology of AIDS: the virus, what it does and how it is transmitted; recognize the role of the host—our bodies—and how we can strengthen our defenses; become wise consumers of medical services by learning to evaluate the risks, benefits, and cost-effectiveness of treatment options; learn to judge wisely and carefully about the things we hear.

PSYCHOLOGICAL—

Understand how AIDS affects our emotions and attitudes, the stress it creates; learn about the resources available to us, and how best to use them; avoid letting fear and anxiety interfere with making sound decisions about our health; recognize the ways in which we are affected by homophobia in society.

SPIRITUAL—

Understand that we are not machines or mechanical beings; our realm of experience goes beyond the physical and some of greatest resources of hope and healing lie in these; recognize that we have a key role in our own healing

SOCIAL—

Understand the key role of love and friendship in our lives, and especially in confronting the AIDS crisis; learn of the tremendous caring and support offered in our community, and learn to become a part of it.

Making choices along that personal path is what this book is about. It won't tell anyone what to do, but instead is designed to provide tools for assessing each person's individual situation and evaluating the available options. Some aspects of healing are well within our range of influence—and some are not. Each of us must develop a personal perspective which integrates the strengths of divergent points of view. This takes considerable effort and willingness to take a hard look at what health really means to us as individuals.

Finally, it's important to recognize that not all viewpoints are of equal value, nor do all have the interests of gay people as their first priority. Science can easily be more concerned with its own advancement or adherence to its traditions than with healing the individual patient. Similarly, many religious, holistic, and mystical approaches ultimately have something to sell—whether it be material products sold for cash, or the institutions themselves which promote their view of the world. You, and only you, can be counted on to have your own personal interests first in mind.

STEPS TO A HEALTHIER FUTURE

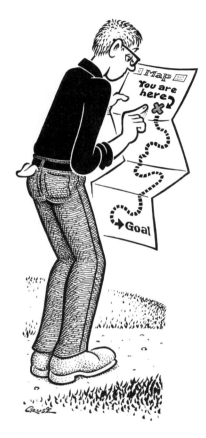

As gay men, we all live with the specter of AIDS. Since first identified in 1981, this deadly disease has spread dramatically. Many of us have friends, lovers, or acquaintances who have been diagnosed with it or died from it. Many of us now test positive to the virus, have AIDS, an AIDS-Related Condition, or signs that our immune systems are not functioning properly. The whole situation is frightening, easily the worst nightmare we've ever faced as a community.

We find ourselves bombarded by stories in the gay and non-gay media which are both depressing and inflammatory. We can't pick up a paper or watch the news without hearing disturbing details about the epidemic or seeing obituaries of its latest victims. We break out in a cold sweat every time a pimple or sore appears. In such an environment, making productive decisions about our health is complicated by the often contradictory information and advice being given. It's all too easy to slip off into despair and anxiety, to feel powerless and hopeless about the future.

Fortunately, there are positive steps we can take to deal with the despair and confusion, steps which can help us develop practical tools to cope with these stressful times. We can learn to separate the truth from the hysteria. We can develop a better understanding of the factors which influence our physical and emotional health. And, if we choose, we can make changes based on this improved understanding.

With so much information and misinformation becoming available about AIDS and health promotion, we frequently become confused and frustrated in our pursuit of personal health:

"Should I stop having sex altogether?"

"What role does diet play? Stress?"

"What about my social life?"

"IS _____ SAFE?" (fill in the blank)

Although no one can answer these questions fully, it is possible to find a personal path to follow. The basic strategies are simple:

- Get the best information you can.

- Assess your situation and develop a reasonable plan of action.

- Get support for carrying out your plan.

- Take action, do something.

Years of accumulated experience with AIDS has shown that people who have a clear and reasonable plan of action are better empowered to face the uncertainties.

Integrated Health Planning

The overall goal of a health strategy depends on your individual situation:

IF YOU ARE WELL BUT WORRIED, your goal might be to reduce the risk of contracting AIDS and to enhance your health.

IF YOU HAVE TESTED POSITIVE TO THE AIDS ANTIBODY, your goal might be to build defenses against the possibility of disease, to minimize the chance of infecting others, and to sort out your feelings on the matter.

IF YOU ARE CURRENTLY ILL WITH AIDS or ARC, your goal might be to learn as much as possible about the illness and your options for confronting it, to learn ways to slow the progress of the disease, to strengthen your body's ability to defend itself, to eliminate the possibility of infecting others, and to come to terms with your own feelings about the situation.

Whatever situation we find ourselves in, we need to develop our ability to lead satisfying lives despite the presence of HIV infection—whether in ourselves or those around us. A comprehensive health plan needs to address at least two key factors which contribute to the AIDS crisis:

• MINIMIZING THE RISK OF EXPOSURE OR EXPOSING OTHERS TO THE AIDS VIRUS

• STRENGTHENING THE BODY'S DEFENSES AGAINST DISEASE

An INTEGRATED HEALTH PLAN can be built upon a simple four-step process:

STEP I: WHERE AM I NOW?
In this step, you examine your current activities and situation to determine the degree of health risk they involve and any opportunities for improvement or desired change.

STEP II: WHERE DO I WANT TO BE?
> Based on self-evaluation, you determine what changes, if any, are necessary and what they should be. In other words, you SET A GOAL for improving your health or minimizing risk.

STEP III: HOW AM I GOING TO GET THERE?
> Once you know where you want to be, you must develop a plan of action for getting there.

STEP IV: HOW DO I IMPLEMENT THE PLAN?
> After making your plan, you have to implement it. As usual, this is easier said than done.

Each of the steps will be examined in greater detail in the remainder of this chapter. Once the concepts are understood, you will be ready to apply them to any of the subjects addressed in later chapters.

**Step I:
Where Am I Now ?**

The first step in an INTEGRATED HEALTH PLAN is to take a look at the current situation. Two questions must be asked:

WHAT AM I DOING?

HOW IS IT AFFECTING MY HEALTH?

In this step, it's important to avoid judgment. The purpose of such an assessment is not to evaluate the morality of our actions. It requires only that we identify what we're doing and to determine whether or how it is affecting our health.

Personal exercises in following chapters will allow this kind of assessment concerning the key issues which affect our health.

**Step II:
Where Do I Want to Be?**

Developing an INTEGRATED HEALTH PLAN requires setting goals to do something about the things in our lives we wish to change. If the self-assessment completed in the first step suggests a need for change in a particular area, we need to set a goal, a description of what we'd like to achieve, what we'd like to do differently, or how we'd like things to be.

A goal is a behavior which can be observed and measured. Here are a few examples:

> *"From now on, I'll insist on using rubbers, whether I'm on top or on the bottom."*

"I'll reduce my alcohol consumption to one drink a day on week-days, two on weekends, beginning with the month of June."

To be effective, a goal must have certain characteristics. It must be:

- REALISTIC AND ACHIEVABLE

- MEASURABLE AND OBSERVABLE

- SET WITHIN TIME LIMITS

REALISTIC AND ACHIEVABLE:
>That is, it must be something we can actually do. If we set lofty "pie in the sky" goals, it may make us feel good for a day or two. But when we inevitably fail at achieving the goals, we feel worse about ourselves than before we started. Any goal we set must be something we can do, something we can live with.

MEASURABLE AND OBSERVABLE:
>It must be something we can describe or see clearly. If a goal isn't measurable and observable, we'll never know when we've achieved it. If we have trouble defining a goal precisely, chances are it isn't measurable or observable.

The two examples of goals given above were measurable and observable. We can easily count the number of drinks, and it's not difficult to know whether we're using a condom or not (sigh...).

SET WITHIN TIME LIMITS
>Setting time limits keeps us from putting it off forever. A goal is meaningless if it doesn't matter when we get around to achieving it. It simply hangs out there like an empty promise or hollow New Year's Resolution. The other characteristics of a goal define WHAT we're going to do. This one determines WHEN we're going to do it.

The two examples given are SET WITHIN TIME LIMITS. Achieving the first goal begins the very next time the person has the opportunity. The second goal begins in June. If the goals were too difficult to achieve all at once, the person might have decided to implement them in stages over a period of time.

A common example of a goal made meaningless by a lack of time limits is that of the cigarette smoker who is always planning to quit—*"any day now"*—but never gets around to it.

Once we set goals, it is important to make a commitment to them. Evidence of this commitment is found in the development of an action plan and, sometimes, in the form of a personal contract we make with ourselves.

**Step III:
How Am I Going to
Get There?**

It would be nice to think that merely stating goals would automatically lead to achieving them, that all it takes is a strong will. Unfortunately, things aren't that simple. Making change is often difficult, particularly in matters as personal and instinctive as our sexuality.

Rather than moving in a single leap from past activities to new goals, it's often necessary to break the goal down into small units or action steps. In effect, we say,

> *"I want to reach this goal. To do so, I'm going to this, that, and the other thing."*

The key concept here is ACTION—the fact that we're going to do some specific thing that will help move toward the goal. We make a commitment to do something that will help, and we stick to it. Sometimes, the action is inherent in the goal itself, while at other times, the goal can be reached by taking a number of smaller steps.

When you set goals in each or any subject areas, you will then have an opportunity to create an action plan for achieving them. Like goals themselves, the actions you plan to take should be written down as commitments you make to yourself or others.

Here a few examples of "action plan" statements that might be included in a health plan:

GOAL #1: Starting today, I will reduce my number of new sexual contacts by half.

ACTION PLAN: Make a list of places in which I'm most likely to make contact for sex; go to them half as often.

Keep track of sexual contacts during the month; know when I'm reaching my self-imposed limit.

Try to have sex more often with fewer people.

GOAL #2: Have safe sex at least once a week without exposing myself to the AIDS virus.

ACTION PLAN: Always carry a pack of rubbers.

Make it clear to my partners that it's safe sex or no sex—before going home with them.

Talk first, play later. Get to know my partners before sex begins.

Make up a *"Safe but Available"* t-shirt. Wear it vainly on the street.

The action plan includes steps which help us move in the direction of the goal. No one of them will allow us to achieve the entire goal, but collectively, they get us moving in ways which make a goal attainable.

**STEP IV:
Implementing the Plan**

Once we set goals and identify action steps, it's helpful to develop a strategy for putting the plan in action. This step deals with the motivation needed to stick to goals and action plans. It's fairly easy to set goals and describe action steps, but far more difficult to motivate ourselves on a day-to-day basis.

A good parallel can be found when someone begins a diet. The goals are usually clear enough and hopefully realistic. The action steps are easy to describe. The diet begins with the best of intentions. Research, however, shows that few people ever succeed in reaching and maintaining their dietary goals on a long-term basis.

Why does dieting so often fail and what can we learn from it?

Diets frequently fail because the motivation isn't strong enough to make the dieter stick to the action plan. The rewards of dieting are too slow in coming to provide much feedback, and the dieter is soon distracted by other priorities. The same thing can easily happen to a health plan. When the health planner is charged up and motivated to take action, the plan seems like a good idea. If that strong motivation diminishes with time, the plan can easily fall by the wayside. Motivation can fade rapidly in the face of new sexual opportunities or frustrations, just as it can when the dieter sees a tempting dessert.

Psychologists have found that people are more likely to keep their commitments to an action plan if they assign CONSEQUENCES. Consequences are what will happen if a person succeeds or fails in keeping an agreement. Motivation to do something, especially something difficult, requires consequences, which may be positive (rewards) or negative (punishment).

For dieters, the image of a trim body may be appealing, but it takes a long time to achieve it. Thus, motivation fades along the way because short-term activities don't seem to produce the desired reward. While avoiding AIDS may be a powerful and important long-term consequence for keeping a commitment to a health plan, it's not very useful as motivator for day-to-day activities. It takes too long to know if you get it, it's difficult to connect to individual activities, and it's too big an item to be effective in motivating short-term, daily activities. *Consequences must be reasonably immediate if they are to work.*

Many people have found that giving oneself a visible, immediate reward for doing something is quite difficult. This takes some practice. Effective consequences should be things which you have control over, such as the following:

POSITIVE CONSEQUENCES:

- See a movie, dinner, a play, a ball game, or concert, alone or with a friend.

- Get a massage, rent that hot new video, phone a 976 number.

- Have a good cry with Judy or Barbra.

- Anything I consider a treat (as long as it's safe).

NEGATIVE CONSEQUENCES:

- No shopping, for days!

- Cancel my subscription to *Drummer* (or *Jock*, *In Touch*, etc.).

- Encourage my friends to go out and have a wonderful time without me (unless that's an inherent contradiction).

Consequences can be as humorous or as serious as we wish. The most effective ones are those which mean the most to us. The more we value our consequences, the easier it will be to reach our goals.

In Conclusion

In the chapters which follow, key risk areas regarding AIDS and health will be discussed. While reading these chapters, you will have the opportunity to develop an INTEGRATED HEALTH PLAN for each aspect of your life which you feel puts you at increased risk of AIDS or endangers your ability to effectively combat it.

Sex and the Gay Identity

Sexual Risk

Rationale for Safer Sex

Getting More, Not Less

CHAPTER

2

SEXUAL PRACTICES

INTRODUCTION

The first aspect of health most gay people choose to examine is sexual activity. This is so not because it's the only thing that matters, but because it has the greatest impact on the risk of contracting AIDS.

Fundamentalist preachers, right-wing politicians and other sexual conservatives, have had a field day with AIDS, using it as a rallying cry against everything this side of the missionary position. AIDS has had little effect on their message—they've always wished we'd crawl back in our closets. Yet now, their message, framed in a chorus of "I told you so's," claims a reasonable-sounding basis in medical science. From their point of view, the only choice left for us is to totally abandon our ways, a choice plainly unacceptable to most of us.

There is another choice—*to learn to live and play safely in the present sexual environment.* The message of this book, and this chapter in particular, is to make it clear that gay people need not surrender one inch of the sexual freedom we've fought for in the past. While AIDS does place limitations on a few sexual practices, it remains possible to lead active sexual lives without endangering our health. One of the longest lasting tragedies of AIDS, and one of the most unnecessary, would be the loss of our hard-won sexual freedoms. AIDS will be with us for many years to come no matter what discoveries emanate from scientific laboratories. It is up to us, the current generation of gay people, to learn to lead our sexual lives in spite of AIDS. It is up to us to see that homophobic preachers and sexual conservatives fail in their twisted exploitation of our suffering.

Sex and the Gay Identity

Concern about AIDS has led to a reversal of the sexual revolution for some, and to a period of self-examination for gay people in general. This is not unhealthy. Even before AIDS, our community suffered great losses from other sexually transmitted diseases, including parasites, syphilis, gonorrhea, hepatitis. With such widespread health problems, there was obviously one aspect of our sexuality we weren't dealing with adequately.

As AIDS awareness has grown, many men have felt a need to change their sexual behavior. Some want to increase safe sexual activities, while others want to decrease activities that risk exposure to the AIDS virus. Making decisions about sexual behavior has been part of our lives since we first became aware that we were gay. Now we face a new challenge:

HOW CAN WE CONTINUE TO BE GAY AND SEXUAL WHILE STILL PROTECTING OURSELVES FROM AIDS?

For some, this seems an almost impossible dilemma. Others have found that it need not be. To put the question into focus, we need to consider what it means to be gay.

IS GAY SOMETHING WE DO OR SOMETHING WE ARE?

It's easy to confuse our gay identity with our sexual practices. So when we consider altering or changing our sexual activities, it's not surprising that we sense a threat to our gay identity. Most gay people experiment with various forms of sexual behavior at different times in their lives, yet continue to be gay while doing so. Thus:

GAY IS MORE THAN WHAT WE DO; IT IS AN IMPORTANT ASPECT OF WHO WE ARE.

Understanding what it means to be gay is a lifelong task. If we look at it this way, we can see that changing our approach to certain sexual activities is not the same as giving up our gay identity.

Conscious and Unconscious Sexuality

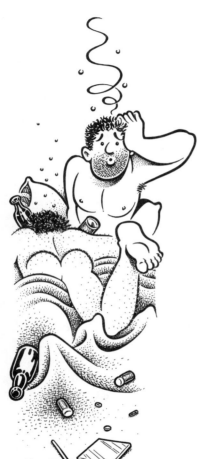

Decisions about sexual activity can be made consciously and under our control or unconsciously and beyond our awareness. When we act spontaneously and go with the flow, *unconscious decision-making* guides our actions. Spontaneity can add excitement to our lives and allows us to break out of our routines and habits, to experience new things. Without it, we might never have explored our gayness at all. But unconscious, spontaneous sexual behavior does not always have pleasant consequences. For example, did you ever wake up in the morning and find yourself looking over in bed at someone and asking,

"How did I GET here?

"Who is THAT?

"What did I DO last night?"

Unconscious choices and spontaneous decision-making have their place. For many of us, much of our sexual experience has been somewhat unconscious, especially in the early years just after coming out. Getting loose, being spontaneous, was a common goal as we developed as gay people. Faced as we are now with a life-threatening disease, careful thinking and planning have a new importance in our lives. By making our decisions about sexual behavior in a clear and conscious manner, we can retain a full measure of sexual satisfaction without endangering our lives.

One of the things that makes sex so wondrous is the experience of being in an altered state of consciousness, being high, not subject to our usual control and inhibition. Sex, often accompanied by drugs, has been the only way for many men to achieve this pleasure. It's not surprising that many find it difficult to change.

AIDS has already been with us for several years, and we will undoubtedly feel its impact for many more. Many men have already learned new ways to achieve sexual satisfaction without endangering their lives. Those of us who haven't must learn soon or face either the loss of our sexual freedom or our health. Restructuring sexual behavior, making it more conscious and deliberate, is a workable choice for all who seek it.

**STEP I:
WHERE AM I NOW?**

The first step in planning to lower the risk of contracting or spreading the AIDS virus and other sexually transmitted diseases is to get a clear picture of our current sexual activities. At the very least, this allows us to raise our risk-taking to a more conscious level.

Most gay people have learned how specific sexual activities incur the risk of infection. While we might expect that our overall risk has lessened, that may not be the case. Although useful information has circulated widely in the community, so has the virus. The risk of encountering people who carry the virus has greatly increased.

Because health risks are affected both by ourselves and by our partners, we must consider two factors: WHAT we're doing and WHOM we're doing it with. WHAT we're doing is the more important because we have clear knowledge of our own activities. With planning and commitment, we can have control over them as well.

Concern over the second issue, WHOM we're doing it with, is easily misunderstood. Early in the epidemic, people believed they were safer if they knew their partners or avoided sex with strangers and people who were very active sexually. If we try to guess whether our partners carry the virus, we will dangerously mislead ourselves.

- Friends and acquaintances are no less likely to be infected than total strangers. The risk might be lower in some parts of the country, but nowhere is it zero. To believe otherwise is to gamble with our lives.

- Unless a person shows visible evidence of infection (typical only in a late stage of disease), there are no legitimate clues based on appearances. "Clean looking" is a worthless predictor of viral status.

- Pre-sex discussions about a potential partner's past exploits are unlikely to be factual if the wrong answers may spoil his plans (especially if he's already turned on).

From the perspective of disease contagion,

When we have sex with one person, we have contact with everyone he has had sex with for the last several years.

And, by implication, with everyone each of his partners had sex with.

Looking for a safe partner is pointless. We must view everyone as a possible carrier. But judgment of another type can play an important role. Although we can't know a partner's health status, we can evaluate his commitment to safe sexual practices. This is the question that we can and should ask:

"Is he willing to play safe and will he respect my limits?"

This should be the question that determines WHOM we have sex with (assuming he passes all the other requirements on our checklist). No moral judgment is necessary or even useful. Sex with many people or with anonymous partners in the past is neither good nor bad. Having lived like a monk or having lived at the baths was a matter of choice, not of moral character (former clerics suggest there's little difference). Now that we know how AIDS is spread, however, we do have moral and ethical responsibilities to each other. Each of us must decide what we will and will not do, with whom and how often we will do them, and whether we need or want to change. We must make these choices consciously and knowledgeably, not out of fear and ignorance.

The first step is to take a candid look at our current activities. Complete the Sexual Practices Inventory that follows.

Sexual Practices Inventory

Instructions:

Estimate how often you engage(d) in each activity on the average, both now and before you became aware of AIDS. Circle which time period you're referring to (Period = times per: W (Week) M (Month) Y (Year)

PART 1 — WHAT AM I DOING?

SEXUAL ACTIVITY	Times per period before I knew about AIDS	Times per period NOW	Period
1. KISSING	☐	☐	W M Y
deep kissing	☐	☐	W M Y
2. MASTURBATION, alone	☐	☐	W M Y
mutual	☐	☐	W M Y
private	☐	☐	W M Y
j/o parties	☐	☐	W M Y
3. ANAL, active	☐	☐	W M Y
passive	☐	☐	W M Y
with condoms	☐	☐	W M Y
4. ORAL, sucking	☐	☐	W M Y
getting sucked	☐	☐	W M Y
swallowing cum	☐	☐	W M Y
5. RIMMING, passive	☐	☐	W M Y
rimming partner	☐	☐	W M Y
6. FISTING, passive	☐	☐	W M Y
active	☐	☐	W M Y
with gloves	☐	☐	W M Y
7. WATER SPORTS, on the body	☐	☐	W M Y
swallowing	☐	☐	W M Y
8. TOYS (dildos, etc.) sharing toys	☐	☐	W M Y
alone	☐	☐	W M Y

43

SEXUAL ACTIVITY	Times per period before I knew about AIDS	Times per period NOW	Period
9. EROTIC MASSAGE --------- ☐ ----------------------- ☐ ------------------- W M Y			
10. OTHER? (List others not mentioned above)			
_____ ☐ ----------------------- ☐ ---------------- W M Y			
_____ ☐ ----------------------- ☐ ---------------- W M Y			

PART 2 — WITH WHOM AM I DOING IT?

SEXUAL ACTIVITY	Times per period before I knew about AIDS	Times per period NOW	Period
1. Monogamous lover			
some or no restrictions ------- ☐ ----------------------- ☐ ------------------ W M Y			
safe sex only ------------------- ☐ ----------------------- ☐ ------------------ W M Y			
2. Non-monogamous lover			
some or no restrictions ------- ☐ ----------------------- ☐ ------------------ W M Y			
safe sex only ------------------- ☐ ----------------------- ☐ ------------------ W M Y			
3. Regular sex partners			
some or no restrictions ------- ☐ ----------------------- ☐ ------------------ W M Y			
safe sex ------------------------- ☐ ----------------------- ☐ ------------------ W M Y			
4. People I'm dating			
some or no restrictions ------- ☐ ----------------------- ☐ ------------------ W M Y			
safe sex ------------------------- ☐ ----------------------- ☐ ------------------ W M Y			
5. Anonymous partners			
some or no restrictions ------- ☐ ----------------------- ☐ ------------------ W M Y			
safe sex only ------------------- ☐ ----------------------- ☐ ------------------ W M Y			
6. OTHERS? (list others not mentioned above)			
_____ ☐ ----------------------- ☐ ---------------- W M Y			
_____ ☐ ----------------------- ☐ ---------------- W M Y			

On Reflection...

As you listed your sexual activities and partners, you might have become aware of your feelings about these matters. The exercise forces you to examine your sexual behavior; it would be unusual not to have some feelings about it. You might conclude that you're having too little sex these days, not enough of the kinds of sex you like, or too much that puts you at risk. Whatever you felt when listing your partners and activities, it's important to pay attention to these feelings.

Now to summarize what you felt after completing the exercise.

THE AMOUNT OF SEX:

☐ I'm not having enough sex anymore
☐ I'm having about the right amount
☐ I'm having too much of the wrong kind
☐ Something else? _____

_____

ABOUT THE KINDS OF SEX I'M HAVING, I FEEL:

☐ Good
☐ Concerned
☐ Worried, scared
☐ Something else? _____

_____

ABOUT WHOM I'M HAVING SEX WITH, I FEEL:

☐ Good
☐ Satisfied
☐ Concerned
☐ Worried, scared
☐ Something else? _____

_____

SEXUAL RISK

To make useful changes in sexual activities, we need to know how the AIDS virus infects people. We've all heard opinions on what's safe and what's not. Some viewpoints seem contradictory and appear to change from time to time. Since AIDS is still a new disease and the research is nowhere near complete, uncertainty will continue. In any sexually transmitted disease, it's difficult to prove that one practice or another is completely safe, or that another is primary culprit. Few if any researchers are testing sexual practices in a laboratory with human subjects and it's unlikely that they will. With this degree of uncertainty, it's hard not to make excuses for our personal favorites.

A lack of absolute certainty is not the same thing as "nobody knows." There are many hard facts about AIDS and sexual behavior. Researchers, including many gay ones who understand and share our interests, are in near unanimous agreement on several points:

- A virus is the principal cause of AIDS; it is now commonly called HIV, or Human Immune Virus.

- Studies have identified body fluids, primarily blood and semen, as the primary medium for carrying this virus between people.

- The virus is most commonly spread by two means: (1) sexual contact which includes the mixing of body fluid (blood or semen) between partners, (2) blood contact through shared use of hypodermic needles in intravenous drug use.

- Undisputed statistical evidence concludes that people who engage in certain sexual activities are more likely to be victims of AIDS; the bottom partner in anal intercourse (the one getting fucked) has the greatest risk of infection. The safety of other sexual acts and positions is less clear.

- As little as a single exposure to the virus can result in infection. Once infected, the virus may well remain with us for life.

Based on this evidence, educational and medical groups have developed guidelines that define the risk of infection. To estimate our own risk, we must take these guidelines into consideration. "Risk" means how much of a gamble we take in certain activities. Researchers warn that no sexual act between two people is guaranteed to be totally safe, but that some are much safer than others. Conversely, some acts place us at much higher risk. The basic rule is simple:

AVOID ACTIVITIES THAT RESULT IN THE EXCHANGE OF SEMEN OR BLOOD, IN ANY WAY, SHAPE OR FORM.

"Safe sex" guidelines apply this rule to specific sexual practices. The Bay Area Physicians for Human Rights (BAPHR, a gay physician's group in San Francisco) provide the following guidelines for evaluating risk. Groups all across the nation provide nearly identical lists.

GUIDELINES FOR SAFER SEX
(from the Bay Area Physicians for Human Rights)

Considered Safe:
Massage, hugging
Mutual masturbation
Social kissing (dry)
Body-to-body rubbing
Voyeurism, exhibitionism, fantasy

Considered Not Safe:
Anal intercourse, no rubber
Blood contact
Vaginal intercourse, no condom
Oral sex, semen in the mouth
Sharing sex toys or needles
Rimming, fisting

Considered Possibly Safe:
French kissing (wet)
Anal intercourse with condom
Vaginal intercourse with condom
Sucking, stop before climax
Cunnilingus
Watersports, external only

(Risk of exposure increases dramatically with multiple partners.)

Rationale for Safer Sex Most of us are already familiar with the safer sex guidelines. Yet several activities remain controversial. Guidelines are just what the title implies—guidelines. The greatest benefit comes not from memorizing the list, but from understanding the whats and whys behind it. Three basic rules provide a quick summary of the guidelines:

• DON'T FUCK WITHOUT A CONDOM

• DON'T TAKE CUM ORALLY

• DON'T SHARE HYPODERMIC NEEDLES OR SEX TOYS THAT HAVE BEEN USED BY ANYONE ELSE.

Most other activities listed as UNSAFE or POSSIBLY SAFE reflect (1) continuing uncertainties by medical researchers, and (2) general health protection. Specifically:

ANAL INTERCOURSE (WITHOUT A CONDOM):
Nearly all relevant studies conclude that anal intercourse places the receptive partner at grave risk. Researchers believe this occurs when infected semen (cum) makes direct contact with blood in the rectum. Man-to-man anal sex often results in some tissue damage, however minor or unnoticed, which causes an opening of blood vessels. Blood need not be visible for this to happen.

Since the virus is known to be present in pre-cum to some degree, withdrawing before orgasm doesn't provide total protection. From a practical viewpoint, we can't always pull out in time anyway, especially under the influence of drugs.

The risk of infection by this route is dramatically reduced by proper use of condoms, especially in combination with spermicides or lubricants which kill the virus. Any intercourse without a condom is unsafe for the passive partner, period. The bottom is at increased risk even if he's already infected, since the act may transmit other diseases which would add to his burden.

For the active partner (top), the risk is not well understood. Infection may require an opening of the skin on the cock, however small, to permit contact with the virus in the rectum. Anal sex with a condom is listed as POSSIBLY SAFE primarily because of the risk of broken condoms. Careful choice and use of lubricants can lower this risk.

ORAL SEX:
Researchers and educators continue to debate the safety of oral sex. Some argue that fluids in the mouth and stomach acids kill the virus in infected semen. Others say that infected semen can easily make contact with blood in the mouth, since open blood flow is common around the teeth and gums. Some counter that since this blood flow is mostly one way—out—it is difficult for the virus to get in.

The statistical evidence is somewhat ambiguous. Some studies warn that virus is present in cum and even in saliva. Recent studies find anal sex carries a much higher degree of risk than oral sex. Some people feel this makes oral sex safe. Careful reading of the research, however, shows that the link to oral sex is not zero, only that it is much lower than that of anal sex. The bottom line? Researchers and gay physicians' groups have debated moving oral sex to the POSSIBLY SAFE category for at least two years. They haven't done so as of this writing. Since safety here is questionable, caution is appropriate.

All the discussions of the risk of infection from pre-cum vs. cum apply here as well. There is a lower concentration of the virus in pre-cum, but it is not entirely absent. Thus the oral sex without cumming falls in the POSSIBLY SAFE category.

KISSING:
Concern over AIDS heightened in 1984 when a researcher isolated the virus in saliva. Later research substantiated this in only a limited number of cases, usually in people with serious opportunistic infections in the mouth or throat. In other situations, the risk of infection through kissing is very minor. Similarly, researchers have found the virus in sweat and tears—in very small concentrations. There isn't a single case of transmission attributed to sweat or tears.

ANAL–ORAL SEX (RIMMING):
Although rimming may not promote transmission of the virus, it is strongly linked to the spread of other sexually transmitted diseases (STDs) like shigella, parasites, and salmonella. All place a serious strain on the immune system, and many AIDS/ARC patients report prior infection with them. Drugs strong enough to treat these infections, such as Flagyl™, are quite toxic and cause distress even to many healthy people. Their use, while necessary, presents an enormous added burden to those who are ill and there are many reports of AIDS and ARC patients whose condition worsened after such treatments. We must consider this indirect risk when making personal decisions about rimming.

Condoms and Lubricants

There is little argument that properly used condoms create a strong protective barrier to the spread of STDs, including AIDS. In 1985, a rigorous laboratory study "simulated" the stress of man-to-man anal sex and concluded that the HIV virus could not pass through condoms (imagine a cluster of doctors huddled together creating this test). Everyone from Sister Boom Boom to the Surgeon General has come out in favor of the use of condoms to prevent spread of AIDS. There is some concern, however, that natural condoms, often made from animal intestines, are not as effective at blocking the virus as latex or rubber-based condoms. Until this question is answered definitively, it only makes sense to stick to the latex.

Lubricants also play a role in this matter. The product used makes an important difference:

THE MAJOR CAUSE OF BROKEN CONDOMS IS THE USE OF OIL-BASED LUBRICANTS (Sorry darling, it isn't because your dick is too big).

Using oil-based lubricants with condoms invites disaster. Only *water-soluble* lubricants (those which dissolve in water) should be used with condoms. Read the labels or ask the local pharmacist. A few well-known brands: K-Y™, LUBRAFAX™, SLIP™, PROBE™, ASTRO-GLIDE™, FOREPLAY™, RAMES™, and LUBRACEPTIC™. To test whether your brand is oil- or water-based, rub some on a finger and run it under cool water. An oil-based lubricant will not dissolve or wash off easily except under hot water or with soap. Water-based products will dissolve easily in any water.

Cleansing Agents

Cleaning up afterward is absolutely no substitute for safe sex. But there are a number of after-the-fact practices that can be helpful. A simple shower can wash away infected semen on the body surface and is a great way to continue the action. Some educators recommend spermicides for use with lubricants and condoms. At least one, Nonoxynol-9, is used because it has shown the ability to kill the HIV virus outside the body. People have used gels, foams and creams for years in conjunction with condoms to protect against sexually transmitted diseases. In recent studies, some products killed the HIV virus on contact. They also can destroy other dangerous microorganisms, such as herpes, gonorrhea, syphilis, CMV, yeast, and trichomonas.

Responsible sex educators, like the Institute for the Advanced Study of Human Sexuality in San Francisco, caution that more research is necessary before they can wholeheartedly recommend use of spermicides. There may be some risk that the spermicides may actually damage the mucosa and thus add to the risk of the virus entering the bloodstream. Spermicides may also give a false sense of protection:

A SPERMICIDE IS NOT A SUBSTITUTE FOR CONDOMS

Instead, they are best used *in conjunction with* condoms.

Sex toys such as dildos that have been inserted in the body must also undergo a thorough cleansing after each use. A simple solution of household bleach, diluted no more than 10 to 1 with water, is an effective HIV killer. This does not suggest, however, that bleach has any role in fighting the virus in an infected person.

With all this in mind, use the tools on the following pages to assess your current level of risk.

Risk Assessment

Instructions:

To evaluate your current risk, you'll need to refer to the activities you listed on the Sexual Practices Inventory (pages 43-44) and compare them with the Safer Sex Guidelines and related explanations.

Before considering your sexual practices individually, first make a rough estimate of the degree of risk you accept in your sexual practices. Circle the number on each of the scales which best describes your risk. Estimate your risk both now and before becoming aware of AIDS.

TOTAL RISK BEFORE BECOMING AWARE OF AIDS

Very low   Very high
1 ----------- 2 ----------- 3 ----------- 4 ----------- 5

CURRENT RISK FROM SEXUAL ACTIVITIES (FROM WHAT I DO NOW)

Very low   Very high
1 ----------- 2 ----------- 3 ----------- 4 ----------- 5

CURRENT RISK FROM PARTNERS (FROM WHOM I DO IT WITH)

No concern for   Complete respect
my limits   for my limits
1 ----------- 2 ----------- 3 ----------- 4 ----------- 5

After doing so, turn to the next page and complete the Sexual Behavior Change worksheet to determine whether you want to make any changes. At this point, you don't need to decide exactly what the changes will be—only the areas in which you see a need for change.

Sexual Behavior Change

Instructions:

This exercise will help you decide which sexual practices you want to change and which you want to continue. There are no right or wrong answers, only your own choices. You alone are responsible for your sexual choices. Make decisions on each of the following:

SEXUAL ACTIVITIES I LIKE BEST:

_____

_____

_____

_____

_____

SEXUAL ACTIVITIES I DO MOST OFTEN:

_____

_____

_____

_____

_____

SEXUAL ACTIVITIES I INSIST ON CONTINUING:

_____

_____

_____

_____

SEXUAL ACTIVITIES I HAVE ALREADY STOPPED OR CUT BACK ON:

_____

_____

_____

_____

_____

SEXUAL ACTIVITIES I WOULD LIKE TO INCREASE:

_____

_____

_____

_____

_____

SEXUAL ACTIVITIES I WOULD LIKE TO STOP OR CHANGE:

_____

_____

_____

_____

_____

Once you have decided which behaviors you want to change, increase, or decrease, you're ready to go on to STEP II to set specific goals.

**STEP II:
WHERE DO I WANT
TO BE?**

Once we've taken a snapshot of our current sexual activities and decided which, if any, changes to make, it's time to establish goals. You may wish to refer to the introductory chapter to review the goal-setting process in detail. The objective here is to develop concrete goals for making any necessary or desired changes in sexual behavior.

Living up to other peoples' rules is difficult, even unacceptable, for most of us. If it weren't, we would all still be in the closet. The ability to cross unreasonable boundaries has allowed us to live our lives freely. Time-worn phrases such as "should and shouldn't," "don't and can't" and "self-control" still ring loudly in our ears. But the fact remains that AIDS and sex are closely connected. We even hear our ourselves and other gay people repeating similar words of caution:

"STOP FUCKING AND SUCKING!"

"FEWER PARTNERS, NO ANONYMOUS SEX!"

"MONOGAMY!" "RELATIONSHIPS!" "ABSTINENCE!"

"YOU CAN'T DO THAT ANYMORE."

"NO! NOT THAT EITHER."

Is this a bad dream? It seems to fly in the face of the freedom we've struggled so long to achieve. Imagine how different the message might sound if our parents had been gay:

"Dear Bruce,

"Loved that hunk you brought home on Sunday! What pecs, what a face, what a ...! If I were twenty years younger you'd have to fight me for him. Isn't he a little old for you anyway?

"We're going out to the island for the week, so have a good time without us. Just remember to play it safe—you know the rules. There's a new pack of 'Skin-tights' by the nightstand, and, please, use your own lube this time—water-based, of course! We both love you so much.

"Love, Dad and Bill."

If our gayness had been affirmed instead of suppressed in our youth, it might be easier for us to accept limits on our sexual behavior now. Before blindly accepting new warnings about our gay behavior, it's important to ask: *"Whose rules are these?"* Do they make sense, are they based on the best information available—or are they just another form of the repression we've been fighting all along? The voices of homophobia often take the lead in demanding that we change, and it's unlikely that their concern is primarily for our safety. When change is necessary, it must be done for our own purposes. There are many worthwhile reasons, including:

- *To lower the risk of contracting illness by sexual transmission.*

- *To lower the risk of transmitting illness to our partner(s).*

- *To relate to others in a different way.*

- *To express commitment in a relationship.*

- *Because we choose to.*

There are at least as many bad reasons. Here are a few that are guaranteed not to provide long-term motivation:

- *To ease feelings of sexual guilt* (see a therapist or join a group instead—there's nothing wrong with gay sex).

- *To get worried family members or friends off your back* (help educate them instead; your sexual behavior is *your* business).

- *To make peace with religion* (religious views on homosexuality are confused, inconsistent, and lacking in scriptural support; homophobia, not spirituality, often motivates our clerical critics).

- *To align yourself with the teachings of the "moral majority"* (you're beyond therapy; consider institutional care).

- *To prepare for a run at the Miss America title* (forget it; *Blueboy* has the pictures *and* the negatives).

Choosing our own sexual behavior is one of the fundamental rights we have fought for throughout history. We needn't surrender it now in the name of good health. When you begin to write out your goals in this section, you'll also be asked to state your reasons or purposes for doing so.

Choosing Goals

Time and reflection are usually needed to set meaningful goals, especially if it's our first try at goal setting. It's most important to select goals that are achievable yet have real consequences. Start by answering a few questions for yourself:

"What change in sexual behavior will most improve my chances of not contracting or spreading the AIDS virus?"

"Do I do anything else that endangers my health?"

A few points to consider when selecting an approach to change:

1. WHAT HAS WORKED FOR YOU IN THE PAST? Have you ever made changes before, and if so, how?

2. WHAT IS YOUR CHANGE STYLE? Confront every change at once, or focus on high-risk behaviors first?

3. WHAT APPROACHES BEST SUIT THE BEHAVIOR you are trying to change? For example, learning to meet new sex partners calls for a different strategy than going cold turkey on a highrisk behavior.

4. BE HONEST WITH YOURSELF.

5. GET FEEDBACK. Ask friends what they think of your plans, or what they have done.

6. TAKE RESPONSIBILITY.

When setting goals, we need to avoid making lofty promises to ourselves that we can't keep—doing so is an effective way to lower self-esteem. At least in this instance, adhering to our goals only some of the time—even most of the time—will not work at all. A single exposure to the virus is all that's required.

Goals and Co-Factors   Is the AIDS virus the only thing we have to worry about? A few other questions to ask when setting goals:

"Why do some people who are exposed to the virus develop AIDS while others do not?" "Why do some people go on living for many years after their diagnosis, others only a short time?"

By now, most of us know there are different forms of HIV illness. Some people seem to develop full-blown AIDS very quickly, while others live on for many years with less severe illnesses. In the early years of the epidemic, we believed that only a small percentage of those infected would develop AIDS. Unfortunately, more recent research shows that the percentage who go on to develop AIDS or ARC grows with each passing year.

What is going on here, and what does it mean to each of us individually? Experts describe two critical factors: (1) the "agent" (the HIV virus) and (2) the "host" (the body and its defense mechanisms). Two people might have similar exposure to the virus, yet one may have greater strength in fighting it. People differ in how long they carry the virus before becoming ill. It's reasonable to believe that the stronger our defenses, the better we are able to fend off disease. Once infected, the longer we can delay progression, the greater the chances of having access to an effective treatment. Anything that blocks infection by the virus or slows its spread in the body will buy time toward the day when a cure becomes available.

Many researchers feel that co-factors play an important role in the course of the disease. Possible co-factors can be any of a wide range of conditions, activities, and substances, including the following:

- CONCURRENT ILLNESSES OR INFECTIONS: outbreaks of several common infections may speed the damage done by AIDS; these include CMV (cytomegalovirus), EB (Epstein-Barr) virus, herpes, and parasites. All create serious added strains on the immune system and some, such as herpes and CMV, may indirectly activate the virus.

- STRESS: stress can weaken our defenses against many illnesses.

- EXERCISE AND NUTRITION: when the body is in top form, its natural defenses are at their best.

- DRUGS AND ALCOHOL: many drugs suppress the immune system. They affect judgment, are commonly a factor in high-risk behavior, and can divert us from proper rest and nutrition.

- EMOTIONAL DISTRESS: severe emotional upset, such as depression or loss of a loved one can lower resistance to illness.

Other chapters of this book discuss some of these co-factors in detail.

Most importantly, we need to pursue goals that will protect ourselves and our partners. All else is icing on the cake. Goals should address avoiding contact with the virus and co-factor infections, and strengthening our resistance to illness.

Goal Setting

Instructions:

- Refer to the Sexual Behavior Change worksheet completed a few pages back. Look at the items you listed under the headings *"Sexual Activities I would Like to Increase"* and *"Sexual Activities I Would Like to Stop or Change."*

- Write goals for changing the factors that most affect your risk of contracting or spreading the virus, or your ability to fight it. Also describe YOUR purpose (not someone else's) for making this change.

- Remember the characteristics of useful goals:

REALISTIC AND ACHIEVABLE
OBSERVABLE AND MEASURABLE
SET WITHIN TIME LIMITS

GOAL #1 (do what?): _____

_____

By when? _____

Your purpose (why?): _____

_____

_____

GOAL #2 (do what?): _____

_____

By when? _____

Your purpose (why?): _____

_____

_____

GOAL #3 (do what?): _____

_____

By when? _____

Your purpose (why?): _____

_____

_____

GOAL #4 (do what?): _____

_____

By when? _____

Your purpose (why?): _____

_____

_____

**STEP III:
HOW AM I GOING TO
GET THERE?**

Once we establish our goals, we need an ACTION PLAN to describe the steps we'll take to achieve them. An action plan for changing sexual behavior should include:

- a description of specific steps or actions;

- the resources we will call on for help (Support from friends? Counseling? Support group feedback? Books? Guides?);

- a way to meet any needs which the previous sexual behavior was fulfilling.

Let's look at each separately.

- SPECIFIC STEPS OR ACTIONS:
These depend entirely on the goal. For example, if the goal is to meet at least one new safe sex partner, we must have a plan for doing so. Where will we go to create the possibility of meeting him? How will we make it clear that safe sex is the agenda? How will we pick him up? (How we will get back in practice?)

If the goal is to always use a rubber when engaging in anal sex, what steps will make that happen? Some possible actions: sample several brands of rubbers and pick a favorite; learn how to use rubbers, alone or with a friend; always carry a pack of rubbers; practice a creative line to use that mentions the "rubber requirement" without turning off a potential partner; practice a line that tells a partner NO when he doesn't want to use one.

The section of this chapter on *"Getting More, Not Less"* describes other possible actions to increase SAFE sexual activities.

- RESOURCES:
These will vary depending on the difficulty of the goal. If the goal is to change long-term unconscious sexual behavior, willpower and good intentions won't suffice, but joining a group or seeing a counselor might. If the goal is to overcome an unreasonable fear of AIDS which is keeping a person locked up at home, one could enlist the help of a friend who hasn't forgotten how to go out and have a good time. Books, pamphlets, and community newspapers are a good source of information. Our community provides abundant sources of help, a fact noted and now envied by many in the straight community.

- A WAY TO MEET OUR NEEDS:
  Sexual behavior patterns are not always random or spontaneous. For many, sex is a means to an end, a way to achieve something else in addition to sexual relief. Sex plays many roles in our lives:

  "Sex is the way I relieve tension and stress."
  (Role: stress relief.)

  "If I don't have sex often, I start feeling ugly and unloved."
  (Role: self-affirmation.)

  "When I'm bored, I can always rely on sex to liven things up."
  (Role: stimulation, excitement, adventure.)

  "Sex is the way I say hello, it's the only way I trust."
  (Role: meeting people.)

Each of these points is valid and real to the speaker. Each might make change difficult if the person chooses to reduce or change his sexual behaviors. For action plans to be realistic, we must determine what, if any, secondary needs our sexual activity is fulfilling. After making changes in sexual behavior, we may also have to find alternative ways of meeting these other needs.

One person above says he uses sex to relieve stress. If he reduces his number of sexual contacts, or limits himself to safe sex, he might find that his stress levels will increase. One solution: learn stress reduction techniques to meet this need while changing his sexual behavior.

Another person says he uses sex to meet people. If he has fewer sexual encounters with new people, he may need to find another way to make new friends. One solution: involvement in community action, support groups, or political work.

When we change something as important as our sexual behavior, we need to look at *all* the things we were getting out of that behavior and find a way to meet those needs. If we don't, attempts to change our sexual behavior will be frustrating and may ultimately fail.

Use the following exercise to describe a personal ACTION PLAN for achieving the goals already established. It might be fun to do this exercise with friends and in a way that allows room for humor.

Action Plan

Instructions:

Refer to the sexual behavior goals you wrote out. Briefly restate each goal below and then develop an ACTION PLAN for achieving it. The plan should include three elements: (1) what ACTION STEPS you will take to make the changes; (2) what RESOURCES you will call on for help, if needed; and (3) what can you do to MEET THE NEEDS the previous behavior was fulfilling.

GOAL #1: _____

Action steps: _____

_____

Resources: _____

_____

Needs the behavior was fulfilling?   How else can you fulfill them?

_____   _____

_____   _____

_____   _____

GOAL #2: _____

Action steps: _____

_____

Resources: _____

_____

Needs the behavior was fulfilling?   How else can you fulfill them?

_____   _____

_____   _____

_____   _____

GOAL #3: _____

Action steps: _____

_____

Resources: _____

_____

Needs the behavior was fulfilling?   How else can you fulfill them?

_____   _____

_____   _____

_____   _____

GOAL #4: _____

Action steps: _____

_____

Resources: _____

_____

Needs the behavior was fulfilling?   How else can you fulfill them?

_____   _____

_____   _____

_____   _____

GETTING MORE, NOT LESS

At this stage of the AIDS epidemic, our community has begun to suffer as much from renewed sexual repression as from any lack of knowledge about safe sexual practices. For many, fear of AIDS and confusion about what's safe has led to celibacy or greatly reduced sexual contact. While this is a perfectly legitimate choice for some, it isn't the only possible answer and it shouldn't be forced on us by others, either directly or through fear of disease.

Sexual conservatives reserve sex exclusively for making babies within legally and religiously sanctioned marriages. Biology and law prevent gay people from meeting that standard, and thus a more liberal view is inherent in our sexuality. Many spiritually-minded gay people find it difficult to believe that an all-knowing, all-powerful, and all-wise God worries about what men are doing with their penises. Surely, there must be greater concerns in the universe.

Sexual activity serves at least three legitimate purposes in our gay culture. It can be:

• an expression of love between partners in a committed relationship (getting it together);

• a response to feelings of sexual attraction felt toward another person, within or outside of a relationship (getting it on);

• a release of sexual urges for personal gratification, with or without strong attraction to an individual (getting off).

If we choose any of these expressions of sexuality, the real moral responsibility we face is to protect our own and our partners' health. Whatever advances medicine may make, AIDS will be with us for many years to come. Other sexually transmitted diseases long pre-existed AIDS and will remain with us long after it. The risk of new AIDS-like viruses will always haunt us because sexual contact is such a fertile ground for transmission of illness. If we choose to retain our right to an active sexuality, the only lasting solution is to learn new approaches that will protect us now and in the future.

Sex, Love and Intimacy

Reexamining our sexual patterns causes us to confront ourselves and the values we've accepted as part of our gay identity. In doing so, many of us find that we weren't completely satisfied with our love lives even before AIDS. For some, sex is easy when it's separated from communication and intimacy. Others are comfortable with intimacy but experience anxiety over sex. Some find both difficult, especially when they come together.

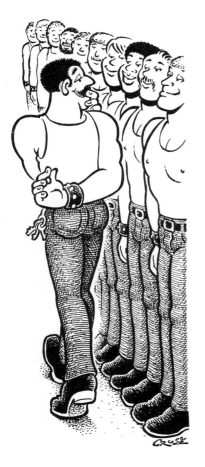

Of course, not all men seek to combine love and sex in the same package. The freedom to have them together or "a la carte" has long been a component of gay liberation. What counts is knowing what we want and pursuing it honestly and openly.

Many men say they welcome a renewed emphasis on the connection between intimacy, emotions and sex. When we choose to explore these deeper issues, we may encounter long-suppressed feelings, such as sadness, joy, fear, and guilt. This can be a good experience as long as we're prepared and willing to deal with whatever comes up. The pressures brought about by AIDS has improved the quality and depth of many gay relationships. This kind of growth, however, doesn't always come easily or without occasional pain. One man put it this way:

> *"I was getting tired of the candy store, but I didn't know how to leave it. I know the problem for me, all right. I'm just plain scared of of getting close. I get jittery. It's intimacy, not sex, that's hard."*

When we seek to get more than sexual gratification out of our relationships, we must expect to put more work into them. That has always been the case. But the threat of AIDS today requires similar additional efforts of us, even if all we want is a good old-fashioned roll in the hay. Once learned, the techniques of increased openness with our partners benefits not only our safety but also the quality of our relationships.

New Tactics, New Strategies

Remember when sex was fun? Even staying within the guidelines for safer sex, erotic, high-intensity action is possible. Just a few practices are completely taboo—unprotected anal sex, and (with considerable debate) oral sex that includes orgasm. The only sacred boundary is the mingling of semen and blood or blood-to-blood contact between partners. Other barriers which are keeping us home alone at night are in our heads, not in the guidelines.

For some, change means little except learning to use rubbers. For those who can't live with rubbers, it might mean learning to eroticize new parts of the body, new acts, or to experiment with more enjoyable forms of masturbation, sex toys, or phone fantasies. Many discover new ways to turn on their partners. Some, through careful and repeated testing and absolute monogamy, create a sexually safe environment in which otherwise "unsafe" behavior becomes possible once again. This method, while attractive, requires careful steps, total commitment, and two antibody negative partners as a starting point.

These approaches are all reasonable solutions for preventing the spread of AIDS. Once we reject those actions that spread the virus, everything else becomes possible. With inventiveness, energy and passion, that leaves a lot of room for play.

For most men, once the facts are dealt with, once the denial and the anger is past, high-risk sex becomes unthinkable, and often, impossible (just can't get it up under those circumstances).

Keeping it safe provides many benefits:

• NO MORE STDS—any of them;

• A POSITIVE OUTLOOK about the future is possible again;

• AN END TO GUILT AND RENEWED ANXIETY caused by failure to play safe;

• A CHANCE TO CELEBRATE OUR SEXUALITY once again.

For those who have found themselves withdrawing from sexuality—against their wishes—a few simple steps can be taken to break loose from the fear and anxiety:

• LEARN (or relearn) both sexual and social techniques;

• PRACTICE—get good at it, relax;

• STEP OUT—no apologies—don't look back; there's a life to live and to get on with.

Sex—gay or straight—is a normal, healthy, and important aspect of human behavior. If we repress it out of unreasonable fears, we suffer individually and as a community.

Attitudes and Rationalizations

Attitudes about safe sex abound within our community and often interfere with our ability to try new approaches. Are these familiar:

"Safe sex is bad sex."

"Safe sex is lite sex."

"Safe sex is boring."

"Safe sex can't be anonymous or spontaneous."

While any of these might be true of a particular sexual experience, none are true as generalities. No one will argue that sex with rubbers is the same as sex without them, but that's a long way from saying that safe sex is always bad sex. Try this test.

> *Would you rather have unsafe sex with a slug (door A) or go to town, using a rubber, on your dream hunk (door B)?*

If you chose the prize behind door B, you've already agreed that some things are more important, more erotic, than direct contact.

We can hold steadfastly to our attitudes—and give up either our sexuality or our health—or we can learn to make safe sex work. If attitude is the problem,

> *"Get off it, girlfriend! YOU'RE the one who's going to lose out."*

Safe sex does lead to more personal contact and a greater sense of intimacy—less anonymity—when we have to communicate with our partner. Yet this very communication might be an enjoyable change from previous sexual habits and sometimes exposes new elements of eroticism we've been missing out on.

On the other side of this coin lies the ever-growing list of

YE OLD FAVORITE RATIONALIZATIONS

"He looks healthy and works out all the time. He's got to be okay." (Appearances tell us nothing about viral status; standards for "looking healthy" diminish in direct proportion to horniness and in inverse proportion to the hour of night.)

"You can't be sure of anything in this world, so I'm not going to change." (Wrong! We know very well how the virus is transmitted; take your head out of the sand before it's buried there under a lily!)

"Rubbers are no guarantee, so why bother." (Rubbers work very well and rarely break unless used with oil-based lubricants; they are vastly safer than going without.)

"I don't believe anything doctors say anymore." (Watch how quickly you change your mind when you suspect you've got a problem.)

"Only the big whores get AIDS. I just get fucked once in a while." (AIDS has no preference for whores (whatever that means); once is all it takes; you've been reading Falwell's pamphlets again, dearie.)

"I went for a psychic reading and so did Steve. She saw long life lines for both of us, so we're going to relax about rubbers." (Is she good at healing too? Better check.)

"Rick and I met last year and have been monogamous ever since—that makes it safe, doesn't it?" (Not exactly; where were you both before last year, and for the last several years before that?)

"He fucked me, sure, but he didn't cum." (You're sure about that? No pre-cum leaked out either, right? You are one sensitive asshole!)

"I just have a real strong feeling that it will be okay just this once." (Could that feeling be coming from your dick instead of your brain?)

"Look, I'm always, always on top." (And your check is in the mail.)

"There's not a chance I'm going to get it." (Perhaps your body should be donated to science; we could use a miracle like this about now.)

"The way I look at it, everybody has to go sometime." (But why now? Think of how much good sex you'll miss.)

"I eat right, take vitamins, work out and sleep peacefully—how could I possibly get sick?" (The same way anyone else can—a virus might enter your body.)

"He's so good looking, such a hunk. I couldn't tell him to put on a rubber. You wouldn't either if you saw him." (Wouldn't it be great to see him again, or let someone else have a crack at him? Did you consider the possibility he might leave if you *don't* suggest a rubber?)

Rationalizations are logical-sounding explanations (often lies) we tell ourselves that no one else would believe. They allow us to avoid facing difficult truths and serve as a form of denial. The "little white lies" we tell ourselves are not harmless when the subject is AIDS. People can argue endlessly to prove rationalizations such as these. What a waste of mental energy! *GET OFF IT!* And get on with learning to live a safe, active life.

Preparing the Environment

Making changes is easier if we prepare the environment to support new activities. Preparations must be made in the first months of an altered sexual style. For example, many people begin with an inventory of sex supplies:

• Toss out all oil-based and Vaseline-like lubricants. Stock up on water-based products.

- Get a spermicide containing Nonoxynol-9.

- Throw out the poppers, all varieties; as long as they're around, someone will use them.

- Have a handy supply of household bleach (for cleaning toys, not your hair, hon).

- Stock up on massage oil or new videos to round out the stash of favorite "props."

One man made up "First AIDS" kits for his friends including Delfen foam (a contraceptive foam with an inserter/syringe), extra rubbers, and Foreplay™ lubricant (with Nonoxynol 9), *"for complete confidence,"* as he put it. His rationale—overdo it. Use rubbers *and* lube with Nonoxynol-9 *and* the foam, so things can proceed without reservation or comment.

Every man owes it to himself to fumble with rubbers in private first. Some practice by jacking off on their own while wearing a condom to get used to the different sensations. At first, it is usual to feel a little like an observer to your own sex life when you go through the *rubber ritual.* Over time, the sense of being a participant returns.

When your approach has been thought out, prepared for, and given a dress rehearsal, your mind can disengage and just follow cues when the lights go down. As a friend said, *"It's hard to keep both your mind and your dick in gear at the same time."*

Confidence increases when we look ahead for possible, predictable crises in keeping safe. Drinking and recreational drugs lower our inhibitions—that's one of the reasons people use them. But they get in the way when learning to be selectively inhibited. Avoid them, at least until new behaviors have become a matter of habit. Certain environments, such as parks, T-rooms, theaters, and baths, are also inappropriate during a learning period. New tricks are best learned at home (or at his home). Most of us have impulsive moments, so we can protect ourselves against moments of carelessness by keeping condoms in a wallet, in the glove comportment, in the gym bag.

Communication During Sex

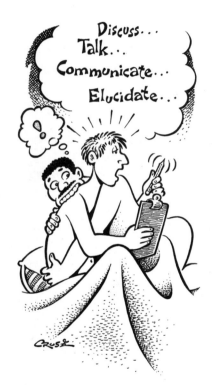

In this new sexual arena, we need new ways to communicate, both verbally and non-verbally. We want to let our partner know that sex must be safe, what our limits are and what we're into. We want to know the same from him. We want to get all this across while still keeping the sexual atmosphere charged up and hot. It may sound like a lot, but it's possible because it's been done before. Men into leather and S & M have long negotiated sex trips in advance with their partners, often anonymously. Two things men seek to manage effectively in these sexual conferences are:

1) Reassurance of sexual interests and limits

2) Mutual, manly respect

Concern over the second part, mutual respect, makes the first part seem more difficult. We fear that raising concerns about safe sex, personal limits and needs, will seem less manly, less macho, less self-assured. Nothing could be farther from the truth. A slender young man with a delicate manner who can express his interests, needs, and limits is more the man than the rugged-looking, unshaven hulk who can only grunt his way through an evening. Manhood has little to do with appearances—that's only the fantasy part. Manhood lies in being able to express ourselves, to stand up for what we want and believe.

A few DO's and DON'Ts for getting the message across:

DO
• Use brief, straightforward phrases.

• Use a cheerful, excited, or lusty tone, to avoid that "too serious" tone that is killer to eroticism.

• Place rubbers and foreplay materials (including a viricidal lubricant) in sight.

DON'T
• Give speeches or lengthy descriptions of your views.

• Bring up your anxieties, fears or AIDS itself, except indirectly (a guaranteed downer with a new person).

• Use medical or clinical terms.

Later, during sex, there may be a need for checkpoints and confirming words. If you don't know each other well, you may expect some misunderstanding, or wonder, *"Did he hear me?"* When they occur, you need to get things clear, quickly and directly. A few examples:

In oral sex, close to orgasm, you might pull back and quickly say:

"Anywhere but in my mouth—I like to watch."

"At the last minute, push my head back and I'll finish you with a firm, wet hand."

"I want to see it fly, Orville."

In other positions, you might find yourself saying:

"Relax. I'm not going to fuck you. I just want to rub and push against your ass."

"Let's switch hands. This one gets so much practice at home."

"Got any water-based lube? I hate that greasy kid stuff."

These examples primarily apply to sex with new men and in cruisy situations where sexual tension needs to be built and maintained. The sex that results will always be more personal than was typical in the seventies. Both partners must be more open and communicative, which leaves some feeling a little more awkward. But many men find they feel more at ease and relaxed for the same reasons.

A lot of men simply now take more time to get to know each other before sex, spelling out preferences and limits. Having such conversations without losing sexual momentum requires a degree of skill, but learning is easy with a little patience and practice. Personal differences play a big role. While one man may feel turned off by talking, another might only get turned on after he feels assured of his safety. Safe-sex negotiations should be handled briefly, put away, and the conversation then turned to more arousing topics.

When using similar approaches with lovers, friends, or regular part-ners, communication should be easier and less threatening. An ex-ception might occur when partners have a regular, unspoken sexual pattern which is risky or unacceptable. This can be just as awkward as talking to strangers. Fear of a partner's reaction, insecurity about his willingness to change can raise concerns about upsetting a good balance in a relationship. The same DOs and DONTs apply, especially if the conversation takes place anytime near the sex itself. Regular or long-term partners can always discuss the details later, making it less likely to lose momentum in a sexually charged moment.

The bottom line for new partners or old lovers is the same: commu-nication is possible and highly beneficial. If we hope to protect our right to a safe and robust sexuality, it is essential.

Feedback

One of the most nagging problems in switching over to safe sex is our self-consciousness about it. We may have spent years learning to be less self-conscious, more spontaneous, more natural in sex with a man. Now, we have to relearn how to be more conscious and deliberate. Of course, there are worse things in this universe than having to practice, one more time, on the sexual playing field.

Most of us learned gay sexual practices one step at a time after we came through the closet door. At first, we knew little about what men did—especially little that was positive. When these mysteries first caught our attention, there were only a few people around to explain them to us. We thanked the stars for aggressive queens, older men, and more daring souls who held our . . . hands along the way. Today, we have greater resources available from the community and our own friends. Juicy conversations with friends can help ease the tension of learning new approaches. A few carefully paced questions should get the ball rolling:

> *"You let him do that?"*
>
> *"He said that to you? And then what . . . ?"*
>
> *"You, Miss Davenport Prim of '68? I don't believe it. I want to hear every last detail. Now."*
>
> *"This is starting to sound like a Harle-queen novel. My own best friend engaged in total debauchery. I love it, and I'm taking notes. Go on. . ."*

We need to listen both to our more conservative friends and our more free-spirited ones. Hearing about their approaches and exploits helps build our own social and sexual skills. But we must hold our own on what's safe and what's not—consensus among friends doesn't change the way that AIDS is spread. If we learn that friends are endangering their lives and those of others, loving disapproval might help clear their heads.

Some men turn to friends or their physician when they find themselves abandoning their goals or feel drawn to unsafe practices. Having an intimate chat with an informed, cautious friend can be very helpful in restoring commitment.

Porn can also be a great teacher. While the actors often take enormous risks, videos can help recharge our sexual batteries and enliven our fantasies—no one has ever been infected by having unsafe sex in his mind. Safesex videos, such as *Lifeguard: The Safe Sex Video* (available from the San Francisco AIDS Foundation) provide an authoritative view on how to do it safely. Books, such as *Safestud* and *Lovesex* by Max Exander (Male), offer a compendium of ways to be both safe and erotic for men who are into leather or want to get back into it in safe ways. Other books, listed in the Resources Appendix of this book, provide step-by-step safe-sex guidance.

The best source of feedback is our partner. We can tell each other what was good and why, and how things could be better next time. Conversation after sex can be frank, friendly and revealing, and is a very important step in integrating new ways. Disappointments and worries can be talked out, helping us overcome the difficulties and strains of the transition. Feedback after sex can be quite erotic, easily leading to the next tumble (practice makes perfect).

Sexual Communication

Instructions:

PART 1: Refer to your list of sexual activities you "would like to increase" or "would like to stop or change" (page 52, 53). Pick out two or three of the most important issues for practice here. Using the space below, write out, in a matter-of-fact and conversational way, what you might say to a partner to tell him what you want or don't want. This is a bit like practicing a new line before using it. Refer to the DOs and DON'Ts described a few pages ago for help.

I want to: " _____

_____

_____

_____ "

I'm not willing to: " _____

_____

_____

_____

_____ "

I want to: " _____

_____

_____

_____ "

I'm not willing to: " _____

_____

_____

_____ "

I want to: " _____

_____

_____
                                                    "
_____

I'm not willing to: " _____

_____

_____

_____
                                                    "

PART 2: Now evaluate the results. Ask yourself how you would respond if someone said these things (what you wrote above) to you. If you don't like the answer,
try doing PART ONE over again—until you develop language that you can live with
yourself.

**STEP IV:
IMPLEMENTING
YOUR PLAN**

Changing sexual behavior can be difficult. Good intentions and new skills are easily forgotten in the heat of the moment, especially when that wondrous condition known as "horniness" sets upon us. It's all quite logical and simple until the pressure of a hard dick— ours or someone else's—enters the picture.

Sex is a mix of friction, fantasy, and surrender. Once we learn to prevent transmission of the virus, the rest is ours. One way to make implementing change easier is to thoroughly indulge ourselves in things that don't put us at risk. Nothing about AIDS restricts our fantasies in any way. If anything, they have become more important than ever. That guy with the crewcut can still become a sailor looking up at you with lonely and oh-so-blue eyes. The boy-next-door type would be so cute fumbling with rubbers "for the first time." The swarthy steel worker who won't cum in your mouth can spray it across your face instead. The big bad guy can still pin your arms to the bed and tell you what to do to make it feel good for him. And you can still want to do it for him.

Pornography plays a big role in fantasy for many of us—magazines, videos, or making your own. It provides a safe and harmless outlet for otherwise unsafe urges. It even gives the Meese Commission plenty of films to watch, making it easier for us to sleep at night. Talking dirty has become a thriving business on the "976" phone lines and provides a useful outlet for unsafe urges. In the bedroom, words and sounds are important for staying in contact with each other in explicit ways. We need to meet the challenge of maximizing pleasure while also maintaining trust. It's difficult to truly let go sexually if we doubt our partner's respect for our limits or his self-control. However explicit we might have been in talking about limits beforehand, verbal and nonverbal cues and directions are still necessary to keep our commitments. Good communication must continue during sex and not be just an aspect of foreplay.

If we are reinventing our sexuality as gay men, it may be a good time to let go of the last of our inhibitions that result from prudishness, religion, or inexperience. We have to avoid a few specific sexual acts—which were often the main course previously—so the next step is to generate as much free space for ourselves everywhere else we can find: in our range of sexual activities, in our capacity for relationships, and talking to other men, and in our ability to love.

Overstepping Our Sexual Limits

In the heat of passion, it's all too easy overstep the boundaries we have set for ourselves. Because the consequences can be so serious, the resulting guilt and discomfort can be overwhelming. People react to this disappointment in different ways. Some decide that sex is too dangerous and avoid it entirely. Some go on living in fear that signs of illness will suddenly appear, viewing each new ache, pain, or pimple in terror. Still others decide engage in the ultimate denial and tell themselves,

"What the hell, everyone has to go sometime."

Guilt and disappointment are especially hard for gay men to experience. Many of us felt guilty about being gay for so long that we now refuse to feel guilty about anything. This is dangerous if we cross the lines of safety.

We need to distinguish between homophobic guilt (guilt feelings imposed on us for being gay) and the discomfort we feel after breaking a personal commitment. Homophobic guilt is inappropriate and we must learn to overcome it. But the disappointment we feel over exceeding our sexual limits can serve as a critical reminder to work harder to protect our health and that of our partners. It's appropriate, even important, to feel disappointed when we cross the lines of safety—our lives are at stake. Yet dwelling endlessly in guilt feelings neither changes what happened nor affects the outcome. The important thing is to learn from our mistakes, renew our commitments, and get on with life.

Consequences and Rewards

To help motivate commitment to our new goals, we can develop a set of possible consequences which we apply to ourself, for ourself. Consequences can be positive (rewards) or negative (penalties). Although AIDS itself is a powerful consequence, its effects only become apparent over the long haul, long after the concern might have done any good. To be effective, consequences must address what happens NOW, tonight, or over the next few days. For example: if the goal is to eliminate an unsafe sexual practice, a possible reward might be more safe action.

Negative consequences or penalties that we assign ourselves serve two important purposes: (1) they are a reminder, a form of feedback that keeps us honest and on track, and (2) they act as guilt containment.

When we exceed our limits, we must take the penalty and get over it, get back on track. Some useful penalties:

- admit the lapse to someone who cares about us (a friend, a counselor, or group);

- give up a legitimate pleasure, such as a weekly movie, a weekend trip or trick, that leather jacket, etc.

When exceeding a limit puts us at increased risk of contracting or spreading the virus, we might try putting in time as a volunteer at an AIDS hospital ward or service bureau. If we learn something from a consequence, all the better.

While assigning penalties may sound like a return to childhood or school days, the effect is quite different when the consequences are self-selected and self-imposed. This isn't a game, after all, this is about our lives and the lives of our friends.

Implementing the Plan

Instructions:

In this last step, list 3 things: (1) any intermediate steps along the way you might use to measure your success in changing sexual behavior, (2) any rewards or consequences you might set for yourself as an incentive, and (3) who you might turn to for help in reaffirming your commitment.

GOAL 1: Steps   _____

_____

Rewards/consequences _____

_____

Who you will turn to: _____

GOAL 2: Steps   _____

_____

Rewards/consequences _____

_____

Who you will turn to: _____

GOAL 3: Steps   _____

_____

Rewards/consequences _____

_____

Who you will turn to: _____

GOAL 4: Steps   _____

_____

Rewards/consequences _____

_____

Who you will turn to: _____

CONCLUSION

The intent of this chapter has been to reaffirm sexual possibilities and re-establish a robust sexuality as one of our options—in spite of AIDS. Some have ignored the implications of AIDS to preserve their sexual freedom, a choice that can only lead to disaster. Abandoning sexuality is likewise a poor long-term solution because it runs counter to our nature. Perhaps we are creating a new world for gay men, one that doesn't revolve around our crotches. For many, this new world has been there all along, but it doesn't require giving up sex.

The epidemic has brought a widening range of emotional experiences into our lives as individuals and as a group. We face fear and sadness, dying and grieving, tending to the sick, and managing our resources for the future. We accept the reality of a witless and hostile governmental reaction to our plight, public hysteria, and new spiritual interests as well as new spiritual attacks. This is what has changed our lives. This is what has altered how we meet and relate to one another and how we play. The social fabric of gay communities in the major cities has changed beyond recognition. All of this affects how we approach sex with each other today. A need for greater thoughtfulness and care has replaced the "do-it-now" party scene, perhaps forever.

Even without effort, we will probably return in time to a robust, eager sexuality. Our sexuality has its own nature and that nature will prevail. This is a transitional period for gay people who lived the sexual revolution. Younger men under twenty-five are coming out in a gay world in which safe sex is the only sex and often have little knowledge of the way things were.

The role of sex, love, intimacy and relationships is under constant reconsideration. Different men, different cities, react at their own speeds based on the local reality of the epidemic. For those who were sexually active before AIDS, a few observations are in order:

- A temporary withdrawal from sex, which may be consciously chosen or spontaneous, is common for many right now and is not, in itself, a problem.

- We can expect a period of confusing or distressing emotional states, often involving anxiety, depression, confusing fears, and anger at doctors or medicine. Sometimes, it will bring our internalized homophobia to the surface in the form of disgust with sex or homosexuality.

- We may have occasional attempts at safe sex that are unsatisfying; likewise, we may experience a reactionary period of unsafe sex, endangering our lives or that of our partners. Practice can solve the problem of clumsy safe sex; renewed and firmer commitments can protect us from future risks.

- After these initial reactions, there often follows a period of better understanding of viral transmission, safe and satisfying sex, our own feelings, and improved relationships.

- A reemergence into sexual life can follow, based on our own tastes, experiences, needs, and decisions.

The sooner we start, the sooner we get there.

What is Stress?

Demands and Resources

Stress Prevention

Stress Reduction

Three Avenues to Relaxation

CHAPTER

3

MANAGING STRESS

INTRODUCTION

Stress has been described in the popular media as the "disease of the 80's." Newspapers and magazines, TV doctors and talk show hosts have made stress a household word. While this popularization has increased public awareness of the impact of stress, it may have distorted the picture by presenting it as the source of all our woes.

Understanding stress is particularly important to gay people facing AIDS. Stress affects (1) our overall health, (2) the functioning of our immune systems, and (3) our decision-making processes.

1. Stress can have a negative impact on our overall health. Research shows that people who experience sustained stress report a wide variety of physical symptoms, including:

    - cardiovascular illness
    - hypertension
    - high blood pressure
    - ulcers & other gastrointestinal difficulties
    - spastic colon

2. Stress is believed to have a direct effect on the immune system. Recent studies have concluded that extended stress can inhibit the immune response to certain types of infection, resulting in greater frequency and severity of disease.

3. Stress can cloud our thinking and decision-making, thus producing indirect effects on our health. People often mistakenly seek relief from stress by increased use of alcohol and drugs or by careless sexual practices.

In an age when our health needs all the help it can get, we need to identify the sources of stress in our lives and take constructive action to prevent or reduce its effects. The link between stress, our overall health, and the immune system is so strong that it's fair to say:

IF WE ARE CONCERNED ABOUT AIDS,
WE NEED TO BE CONCERNED ABOUT STRESS.

What is Stress?

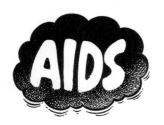

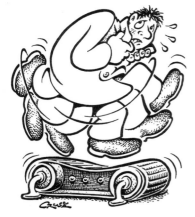

Stress itself is not a disease, nor is it transmitted by bacteria or viruses. Yet, it is a factor in numerous diseases, including AIDS. To better understand stress, we need to define it and its components. Unfortunately, popular attention has blurred the definitions, lumping all aspects of the condition simplistically under the term "stress." This book will use the following terms and definitions:

STRESS:
    A feeling of tension or pressure experienced when we feel that the DEMANDS placed on us are greater than the RESOURCES we have available to meet them.

STRESSORS:
    The events, situations, or demands which we PERCEIVE to be the sources of stress.

STRESS RESPONSE:
    The instinctive, biological reactions our body makes when confronted with stress.

COPING RESPONSES:
    The actions we take to try to cope with stress. These include both actions and thoughts. Not all coping responses are effective in reducing the stress response. Some, such as the use of alcohol and drugs, often increase the STRESS RESPONSE.

DEMANDS can be internal or external:

INTERNAL DEMANDS include our needs, expectations, personal standards, past history. (*"I must look absolutely flawless or I'm not going to the party. My public expects it of me."*)

EXTERNAL DEMANDS include other peoples' needs and expectations, changes or events which affect our home life, work, or community. (*"If you spend the evening flirting with everyone else at the party, you'll need a new address by dawn."*)

RESOURCES can also be internal or external:

INTERNAL RESOURCES include our own abilities, attitudes, skills, and values. (*"Listen doll, I may not be as young as I used to be, but I can handle myself. One icy stare from these eyes and I'll cut through that crowd like Moses through the Red sea."*)

EXTERNAL RESOURCES include friends, lovers, money, and any material or equipment which might be called upon to meet demands. (*"No need to fret, love bunch. I'll loan you some jewelry. Remember that glitzy chain and the two bracelets I bought? They'll keep us within two feet of each other all night."*)

Stress occurs when we perceive that our RESOURCES are inadequate to meet the DEMANDS that stressors place on us.

Stress and Perception

Although stressors and demands in our lives are very real, the degree to which they result in stress is dependent on our perceptions. The more we PERCEIVE or believe that demands exceed our available resources, the more stress we experience. The more stress we experience, the stronger the stress response triggered in our bodies. Two people can experience the same situation but perceive it differently. One may be stressed out by it, while another may be able to laugh it off. Consider the following example:

Two guys sit down in a bar. Both see an attractive stranger sit down nearby, and both catch his eye for a moment. One sees the situation as an opportunity and experiences just enough stress to perk up from the indifferent mood he had felt before the stranger walked in. For him, this modest amount of stress helps bring out his best and makes it possible for him to start a conversation. The other guy feels very insecure, perceiving that the stranger is out of his league and couldn't possibly be interested in him. In other words, he feels his resources aren't up to the demand. This higher degree of stress may lead him to feel tense, break out in a nervous sweat, or even withdraw. Despite the differences in response, both are responding to the same situation, namely, a handsome stranger—whose real interests or tastes are unknown to both of them.

Shifts in our perception can thus be a key to reducing stress.

The Importance of Stress

Stress itself is a fact of life that will never disappear completely—nor should it. It is only when stress becomes excessive or prolonged that problems arise. The stress response is one of the body's ways of defending itself. Without it, we would never have survived the trials of evolution. Stress prepares the body to respond to demanding or dangerous situations. When a person is confronted with a dangerous situation, the stress response prepares him to either fight or retreat. In our own lives, we all experience the stress response:

Have you ever been confronted by "fag-bashers" or muggers?

Have you ever prepared for an important athletic event, a speech, or a contest?

Have you ever sat down at a business dinner and had your boss ask you when you're going to get married?

Have you ever tried to make a date with a man who was so hot that you were afraid you just didn't have a chance?

Think of how you felt—physically—in these situations. Your heart raced, your palms became sweaty, muscles tensed in your arms and legs, your stomach knotted. These weren't figments of your imagination, but real, physical events brought on by changes in body chemistry. Other less noticeable effects may have included changes in breathing, dilation of the pupils, narrowing of attention, and a pause in digestion. These responses to stress are universal and predictable. They sound and feel a lot like the changes experienced under the influence of a powerful drug, illness, or medication.

Although the stress response evolved as a protective measure, it can also work against us. When constantly confronted with demands and inadequate resources, we experience CHRONIC STRESS: a nearly constant state of the stress response, constant preparation for battle. The resulting change in body chemistry has been linked with many disorders. Many of us experience CHRONIC STRESS in our response to the AIDS crisis.

Each of us has an optimal level of stress which permits us to operate at peak capacity. The stress of city life might create chronic stress for one person, while barely keeping a New Yorker awake. Our tolerance for stress varies from time to time and its effects appear to be accumulative. Weekends, vacations, and time off are needed to allow a healthy escape from everyday demands. If we endlessly take on one challenge after the next, we inevitably encounter a crisis, ranging from simple burnout to a total nervous breakdown.

At the other extreme, the total absence of stress can lead to terminal boredom. When life presents nothing more taxing than the choice of which beach to lie on, most people become restless (well, perhaps after a month or so). In *Stress Without Distress,* Hans Selye suggests that stressors are challenges. Meeting challenges—especially those which we feel are worthwhile—gives our lives meaning. We grow and learn from our experience of overcoming new obstacles.

When fighting an HIV infection, maintaining a balance between living a meaningful life and not suffering the effects of prolonged stress can be a real challenge. Withdrawal from all demands might sound attractive, but if it takes away all meaning, all excitement and interests in life, it will do more harm than good. Without accepting challenge or some willingness to face demands, we lose the will to live. For those who are ill, deciding how to best use limited energies and resources is a critical choice that deserves careful consideration.

Unraveling Stress

The feeling of being overwhelmed by stress is all too common for gay people. In our earliest days, we lived with the fear of knowing we were different, and that our hidden difference stirred feelings of anger and disgust among friends, family, and society. Demands were placed on us to be like everyone else. We couldn't because we weren't, and we felt very alone. Thus, we faced one of our first experiences of a demand we didn't have the resources to handle.

If we came out as teenagers, we had to confront the hostility and bigotry of others. Much of it became internalized and we found it difficult to love or accept ourselves. We were shunned for being different and we weren't even very sure that we liked ourselves. We perceived demands we didn't have the resources to handle. We envied straight friends whose biggest concerns seemed to be acne and learning to dance (they're *still* working on that one).

As adults, many of us found acceptance among gay friends, in our community, and, for some, with our families. We learned the fine art of picking-up and the closing-hour shuffle. And then, just when we thought we knew it all, we encounter a deadly disease running rampant in our community. Our sexual freedom is again restricted, our friends are ill or dying, and it seems like the rest of society doesn't care. Instead of the joys of having arrived, we're now facing crises usually associated with old age. Once again, we perceive demands we feel we don't have the resources to handle.

For those who have fallen ill, the demands reach new heights:

- compounding financial troubles
- confusion over medical choices
- shattered dreams, fear of death
- loss of employment
- loss of friends and lovers
- forced coming out, exposure
- well-meaning but clumsy efforts to help
- condemnation by religious groups.

As gay men we experience stress in three key aspects of our lives:

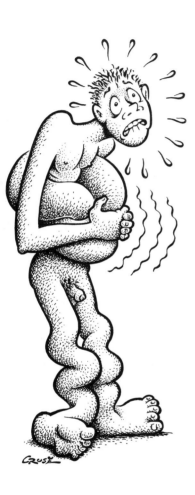

1. STRESS OF EVERYDAY LIVING:
   The responsibilities of living and working in a world where rapid changes place constant demands on us (gay people have to worry about waxy yellow buildup just like everyone else).

2. STRESS OF BEING GAY IN A HOMOPHOBIC WORLD:
   Outside of a few enclaves, we're not exactly the dominant species. In addition to a hostile environment, we each have our own internalized homophobia which can easily work its way to the surface. This results in strong internal tension and often disrupts our relationships with other gay men.

3. STRESS OF THE AIDS CRISIS ITSELF:
   You want to know about stress? Talk to a gay man about AIDS. The crisis forces us to confront ourselves and our mortality. We face sorrow, anger, and profound loss when we least expect it and are perhaps least equipped to handle it.

On the bright side, we have learned there is ample understanding, love, and joy (resources) in our community to meet these demands. AIDS has truly brought out the best in us along with all the pain. Although there are no quick solutions, we can increase our awareness of the sources of stress in our lives and work to develop effective ways to cope with them. To examine how each of these areas may be affecting you as an individual, take a few minutes to complete the exercise on the following pages.

Demands and Resources

Instructions:

List some of the major demands which you currently experience in each of the three key areas. Pay particular attention to demands placed on you related to the AIDS crisis. List the internal and external demands separately. Then list the resources you feel you have to respond to the demands.

1. THE STRESS OF EVERYDAY LIVING

    Internal DEMANDS (needs, expectations, personal standards, past history)

    _____

    _____

    _____

    _____

    Internal RESOURCES (abilities, attitudes, skills, and values)

    _____

    _____

    _____

    _____

    External DEMANDS (other peoples' needs and expectations, changes or events)

    _____

    _____

    _____

    _____

    External RESOURCES (friends, lovers, money, and any material or equipment)

    _____

    _____

    _____

    _____

2. THE STRESS OF BEING GAY IN A HOMOPHOBIC WORLD

    Internal DEMANDS

    _____

    _____

    _____

    _____

    Internal RESOURCES

    _____

    _____

    _____

    _____

External DEMANDS

_____

_____

_____

_____

External RESOURCES

_____

_____

_____

_____

3. THE SPECIAL STRESS OF THE AIDS CRISIS

Internal DEMANDS

_____

_____

_____

_____

Internal RESOURCES

_____

_____

_____

_____

External DEMANDS

_____

_____

_____

_____

External RESOURCES

_____

_____

_____

_____

SUMMARY:

Based on the reflections above, I feel:

☐ Overwhelmed; demands far outweigh my resources.

☐ Challenged by stress, but I have strong resources.

☐ I've got things pretty well under control.

☐ Gay as a daisy and this is all so silly.

**STEP I:
WHERE AM I NOW?**

It's not enough to simply talk about stress. The objective of stress management is to DO something about it. Coping responses, the things we do about stress, attempt to change the balance between demands and resources, either by eliminating or modifying the demands, or by increasing the resources available for meeting them. Coping responses include actions that help us avoid becoming overly stressed and things we can do to directly reduce the stress we experience. The more effective our coping responses, the better we are able to manage stress. Using a step-by-step, planned approach can make it possible to combat stress at the source, as well as give us tools for handling the kinds of stress we all must live with.

As a starting point, we need to estimate the amount of stress we are currently facing. We can do this in at least two ways:

1. Identify and add up the STRESSORS (sources of STRESS) we are experiencing.

2. Identify the STRESS SYMPTOMS we are experiencing (physical symptoms which might be the result of stress).

Research has shown that one way to understand the level of stress we experience is to look at the number and nature of changes that were required of us in one year. These events are sometimes called "stress triggers." Research shows that the more changes are required of us, the greater the likelihood that we will experience stress and become ill. One widely used research tool uses a scale to measure the level of stress experienced by a person in one year.

An example of this type of scale, adapted for gay people confronting AIDS, is found on the next pages. Use it to estimate the amount of stress you've faced in your life during the last year.

A second scale is provided for noting the signs of stress response which you are experiencing. Using both scales will give the broadest picture of your current level of stress.

Stressors in the Past Year

Instructions, Part One:

1. CHECK OFF EACH OF THE EVENTS WHICH YOU HAVE EXPERI-ENCED within the last year, in each of the 3 categories. You may interpret the word family to mean your closest circle of friends (your extended family) as well as your biological family.

2. ESTIMATE THE DEGREE OF STRESS you feel each event is causing you; use the numbers on the scale below to determine your ratings:

Just a little		Some		A great deal
1 ----------	2 -----------	3 -----------	4 ----------	5

For the moment, IGNORE THE "A B C" COLUMN AT THE FAR RIGHT under the heading GROUP. This part will be used in a later step.

Stressors Assessment Scale

THE STRESS OF EVERYDAY LIVING (assume all are for non-AIDS, non-homophobic reasons):

Event	Estimate	Group		
Death of your lover	☐	A	B	C
Permanent breakup with lover	☐	A	B	C
Separation from lover	☐	A	B	C
Jail term	☐	A	B	C
Death of close family member	☐	A	B	C
Personal injury or illness	☐	A	B	C
Start a new intimate relationship	☐	A	B	C
Fired from work	☐	A	B	C
Reconciliation with lover	☐	A	B	C
Retirement	☐	A	B	C
Change in close family member's health	☐	A	B	C
Sexual difficulties	☐	A	B	C
Major change at work	☐	A	B	C
Change in financial status	☐	A	B	C
Death of a close friend	☐	A	B	C
Change to a different line of work	☐	A	B	C
Change in the number of arguments with you lover	☐	A	B	C

Event	Estimate	Group		
Mortgage, loan, or debts over $10,000	☐	A	B	C
Foreclosure of mortgage or loan	☐	A	B	C
Change in work responsibilities	☐	A	B	C
Son or daughter leaving home	☐	A	B	C
Trouble with family members	☐	A	B	C
Outstanding personal achievement	☐	A	B	C
Spouse begins or stops work	☐	A	B	C
Starting or finishing school	☐	A	B	C
Change in living conditions	☐	A	B	C
Trouble with boss	☐	A	B	C
Change in work hours, conditions	☐	A	B	C
Change in residence	☐	A	B	C
Change in schools	☐	A	B	C
Change in recreational habits	☐	A	B	C
Change in church activities	☐	A	B	C
Change in social activities	☐	A	B	C
Mortgage, loan, or debts under $10,000	☐	A	B	C
Change in sleeping habits	☐	A	B	C
Change in number of family gatherings	☐	A	B	C
Vacation	☐	A	B	C
Christmas/holiday season	☐	A	B	C
Minor violation of the law	☐	A	B	C

(Now add the scores)

MY STRESSORS SCORE in this category .... _____

THE STRESS OF BEING GAY IN A HOMOPHOBIC WORLD (assume all are for homophobic reasons, including internalized homophobia—your own):

Event	Estimate	Group		
Rejection by family or friends	☐	A	B	C
Jail term	☐	A	B	C
Police harassment	☐	A	B	C
Personal injury or illness (fag bashing)	☐	A	B	C
Sexual difficulties	☐	A	B	C
Fired from work	☐	A	B	C
Major change at work	☐	A	B	C
Change in financial status	☐	A	B	C
Change to a different line of work	☐	A	B	C
Change in the number of arguments with your lover	☐	A	B	C
Foreclosure of mortgage or loan	☐	A	B	C
Change in work responsibilities	☐	A	B	C

Event	Estimate	Group		
Trouble with boss	☐	A	B	C
Son or daughter leaving home	☐	A	B	C
Trouble with family members	☐	A	B	C
Change in living conditions	☐	A	B	C
Revision of personal habits	☐	A	B	C
Change in work hours, conditions	☐	A	B	C
Change in residence	☐	A	B	C
Change in schools	☐	A	B	C
Change in recreational habits	☐	A	B	C
Change in church activities	☐	A	B	C
Change in social activities	☐	A	B	C
Change in sleeping habits	☐	A	B	C
Change in number of family gatherings	☐	A	B	C

(Now add the scores)
MY STRESSORS SCORE in this category .... _____

THE STRESS OF THE AIDS CRISIS (assume all are for AIDS-related reasons):

Event	Estimate	Group		
Death of your lover from AIDS	☐	A	B	C
Lover sick with AIDS	☐	A	B	C
Lover sick with ARC	☐	A	B	C
Lover tested positive to AIDS antibody	☐	A	B	C
Permanent breakup with lover	☐	A	B	C
Separation from lover	☐	A	B	C
Personally ill with AIDS	☐	A	B	C
Personally ill with ARC	☐	A	B	C
Personally tested positive to AIDS antibody	☐	A	B	C
Fear of contracting AIDS	☐	A	B	C
Death of close family member	☐	A	B	C
Start a new intimate relationship	☐	A	B	C
Change in the number of arguments with your lover	☐	A	B	C
Change in close family member's health	☐	A	B	C
Sexual difficulties	☐	A	B	C
Reduction in cherished sexual practices	☐	A	B	C
Fired from work	☐	A	B	C
Change to a different line of work......................................	☐	A	B	C
Change in financial status	☐	A	B	C
Change in work responsibilities	☐	A	B	C

(Now add the scores)
MY STRESSORS SCORE for this category .... _____

3. TOTAL YOUR OVERALL SCORE by adding up the total scores for each of the three categories.

   MY COMBINED TOTAL STRESSORS SCORE .... _____

4. AFTER REFLECTING ON THIS EXERCISE, I FEEL:

   ☐ I'm less stressed than Twiggy's bra—no problem, my health isn't threatened.

   ☐ About the way the Marine's felt when the fearsome army of Grenada counter-attacked—some stress, but not enough to be alarmed about.

   ☐ I ought to keep my fingers crossed;

   ☐ It's been a hell of a year; if I'm not sick now, it's a miracle.

   ☐ I'm entitled to a nervous breakdown; it's mine, I earned it, I feel it coming; (and I better do something about it).

Before beginning with step 5, take a brief rest from all this introspection. Otherwise, this exercise itself might wind up on your list of STRESSORS.

5. Now go back over the entire list (really!). In the column at the far right, along side each of the STRESSORS you are experiencing, circle A, B, or C to describe which category it best fits into:

   GROUP A: Stressful situations or STRESSORS which will take care of themselves, get better, or pass with time, regardless of what I do about them.

   GROUP B: Stressful situations or STRESSORS which I might be able to do something about.

   GROUP C: Stressful situations or STRESSORS which feel I can't do anything about and will have to endure.

Stress Symptoms

Instructions, Part Two:

1. INDICATE WHICH OF THE FOLLOWING SYMPTOMS YOU HAVE EX-
PERIENCED in the past year by placing a check mark in the box alongside the
symptom. Research has shown that all may be linked to chronic stress.

Symptoms

Column A	Column B*
☐ Muscular tension	☐ High blood pressure
☐ Headaches	☐ Chronic constipation
☐ Backaches, neckaches	☐ Irritable bowel
☐ Sexual problems	☐ Chronic diarrhea
☐ Indigestion	☐ Ulcers
☐ Muscle spasms	☐ Insomnia
☐ Anger, hostility	☐ Suicide thoughts/attempts
☐ Fears	☐ Obsessions, unwanted thoughts
☐ Fatigue	☐ Phobias/panic
☐ Sleeping difficulties	☐ Depression
☐ Dizziness	☐ Anorexia or obesity
☐ Resentment, Irritability	
☐ Others?	
☐ _____	
☐ _____	

NOTE: Any of these symptoms may also have physical causes. You should have a
medical doctor eliminate the possibility of such problems before assuming that your
symptoms are solely stress-related.

*COLUMN B symptoms are serious conditions which demand medical attention,
regardless of their cause. You may also wish to consult a professional trained in
stress management.

2. Of the STRESS SYMPTOMS you identified above, list below those which you are most concerned with.

_____   _____

_____   _____

_____   _____

_____   _____

_____   _____

_____   _____

2. AFTER REFLECTING ON THE ABOVE, I FEEL:

☐ Fortunate to be as healthy as I am.

☐ Some evidence of stress, but not enough to be alarmed about.

☐ Considerable evidence of stress and need to understand it better.

☐ Either I'm a hypochondriac or stress is doing me in; it all makes sense now. . . . yeah, that's it.

☐ Like going to bed for a month.

**STEP II:
WHERE DO I
WANT TO BE?**

Some degree of stress is present and necessary in everyone's life. In the age of AIDS, stress carries a heavier burden than usual. Not only is stress more likely, but research indicates that excessive stress may have a direct role in suppressing the immune system. This further complicates the problem for those who are ill.

While not all stress can or should be eliminated, a good portion of it, and its effects, can be managed. The first step was learning about the stress factors in your present life. In the second step, you make decisions about where you'd like to reduce the stress in your life. When analysis of the stress factors and stress responses in our lives suggests a need for change, it's time to set goals. Targets for change must be reasonable and achievable. Eliminating all stress is neither desirable nor possible. The first stage of goal setting, therefore, is to establish priorities so that we can focus our goals and stress management efforts on things we can actually do something about.

Based on the insights gained in the previous exercises, complete the two parts of goal-setting exercise on the following page.

Setting Goals

Instructions, Part One:

The STRESSORS you labelled as group B and C are good targets for goal setting since they are things you can do something about or have to endure. Likewise, the STRESS SYMPTOMS you identified are important indicators that you need to do something about stress. Ignoring them can cause you harm.

Keeping in mind the qualities of a good goal, set at least two goals related to the stress in your life, two things you'd like to accomplish regarding your STRESSORS or STRESS SYMPTOMS. For now, you needn't be concerned about HOW you're going to do it, but only WHAT you want to change. For EXAMPLE:

By September of this year, I'd like to reduce or eliminate (headaches?) (neckaches?) I'm experiencing as a result of stress.

Before the end of the month, I will end or restructure that unproductive relationship I'm hanging on to (the one causing me to turn gray before my time).

Finally, for each GOAL, describe your purpose, or what you hope to accomplish by achieving this goal.

GOAL 1 (CHANGE WHAT?): _____

_____

BY WHEN? _____

YOUR PURPOSE (WHY?): _____

_____

GOAL 2 (CHANGE WHAT?): _____

_____

BY WHEN? _____

YOUR PURPOSE (WHY?): _____

_____

**STEP III:
HOW AM I GOING
TO GET THERE?**

There are two general strategies for managing stress:

STRESS PREVENTION: Actions which help us avoid stress in the first place. Stress prevention focuses on efforts to reduce the demands we face, through problem-solving, altered decision-making, or changes in the environment itself.

> EXAMPLE: Bill got stressed out at the glitzy discos he was attracted to. All the youthful energy, sweaty muscles, and practiced attitude shook his knees and wilted his weenie.
>
> A *stress prevention* solution: he tried going to a neighborhood bar instead. To his surprise, he discovered a hot crowd hungry for new faces and a whole lot less attitude. No more Saturday night stress, and a new star was born on 14th Street.

STRESS REDUCTION: Actions which reduce the impact of stress by inhibiting or minimizing the stress response. These include breathing exercises, meditation, and visualization.

> EXAMPLE: Terry shared Bill's dance bar anxiety but was drawn to the scene like TV preachers are to other people's money. If he could only quell the shaking, hyperventilation, and indigestion, he was sure he would get with it any day now.
>
> A *stress reduction* solution: a monk he met in the john signed him up for a Karma Mantra meditation class, where he learned a great relaxation routine and a few breathing exercises. He used them before, during, and after the bar to ease his inner turmoil. Last week, he placed second in the wet jockey shorts contest and took the winner home with him.

While either strategy can help reach our goals, neither is a panacea for all our problems. Often, the situation itself will call for one approach or the other. When the factors causing stress are within our control, as was the case in the examples above, either stress prevention or stress reduction is possible and largely a matter of personal preference. If the source of stress is something we have no control over and must live with, only stress reduction may be possible.

Stress Prevention

Stress prevention is frequently overlooked, perhaps because it is difficult to package or commercialize. No matter how proficient we become with stress reduction techniques, our ability to reduce the stress response is limited. If we continually create or place ourselves in stressful situations, stress will eventually overwhelm us. Preventing stress requires a careful assessment of the demands we face, why we are facing them, and what resources we are using to meet them. We must ask: *Are the demands necessary and unavoidable or are they self-imposed? What happens if they are not met?*

We are not mere victims of fate. Many demands we feel are of our own doing—and thus subject to our undoing. Demands imposed by self-chosen career or income goals, or a desire to out-flash the neighbors are entirely within our control. Those who are ill often report how difficult it is to let go of such demands, even when necessary.

Our decision-making can also be a major contributor to stress. Demands which come from our inner voices and personal standards can be very stubborn since we aren't always aware of the extent of their influence on us. For example, consider the plight of Tillie, a once and future Empress of a great farm state:

> *Tillie prided herself on her high standards of grooming. Her mother had always told her "If you don't have your looks, you don't have anything." Tillie lived this credo and vowed not be seen in public except when at her near perfect best. How else could one be a worthy Empress? As the years passed, such moments of perfection came fewer and farther between. Outings required days, not hours, of preparation, yet Tillie simply wouldn't violate her standards. What would her public say? The mere thought of going out made her faint. She knew just how Queen Elizabeth must have felt all those years.*

> *Increasingly isolated and self-conscious, Tillie was no longer a well woman. But, with effort, friends convinced her to reconsider the demands she had created for herself, to forgo mother's warnings which still echoed in her ears. Tillie eventually realized that she was loved with or without mascara and re-emerged as a less stressed, if aging, goddess.*

Like Tillie, we must examine the degree to which our own choices and decisions have created or added to the demands we face. Fortunately, what we do, we can undo. Decision-making works in both ways—it can help us prevent stress as well as produce it. By rethinking decisions and personal choices which contribute to stress, we can change the balance of demands and resources in our favor.

Use the exercise on the following pages to recognize any decisions you've made which might contribute to your own level of stress.

Decision-Making and Stress

Instructions:

In the space below, describe an important situation in your life which is causing stress, preferably one of the STRESS FACTORS you labelled as GROUP B on pages 91-93. Ask yourself each of the following questions about the situation.

STRESSFUL SITUATION: _____

How does the stress become apparent? _____

_____

What am I trying to accomplish in this situation? _____

_____

_____

Is my goal or objective in this situation reasonable? _____

_____

What choices or decisions have I made which contribute to the stress? _____

_____

_____

Is there another way to accomplish what I want, one that might result in fewer demands, or less stress? Describe it if possible. _____

_____

_____

The Six A's of Change

Our ability to prevent stress is not limited to undoing our own decisions. Although some of the things which cause stress in our lives are not our of own doing, we do have options regarding how we respond to them. Before passively accepting stress, we can ask a few simple questions which help us explore the options. The six questions:

1. What can I **A**void?

2. What can I **A**lter?

3. What can I **A**dapt?

4. What are my **A**lternatives?

5. What can I **A**ccept and enjoy?

6. When will I take **A**ction?

The questions can be asked of any stressor, whether caused by our internal decision-making or by external demands. There's no magic to the formula—it's just an easy way to remember the right questions to ask. When applied to important stressors, the six questions help us set priorities, decide what to let go of, and what we can make better use of. The objective, as in all stress management efforts, is to change the perceived imbalance between demands and resources.

Take the time to apply this concept in developing an action plan for stress prevention. Later, a second part of the action plan will be directed toward reducing the impact of stress from those stressors which don't yield to stress prevention.

Action Plan—Prevention

Instructions:

Select what you feel is one of your most significant STRESSORS from those you labelled as Group B (those which you can do something about) in the exercise on pages 91-93. Ask yourself the Six A's about this stressor.

This process can, and should, be repeated for each of the major STRESSORS you wish to do something about.

Concerning an important GROUP B STRESSOR:

1. What can I AVOID? _____

_____

2. What can I ALTER? _____

_____

3. What can I ADAPT? _____

_____

4. What are my ALTERNATIVES? _____

_____

5. What can I ACCEPT and enjoy? _____

_____

6. When will I take ACTION? _____

_____

Stress Reduction: Three Avenues to Relaxation

Stress prevention can seldom provide the entire solution since we don't have control over all the events which cause stress. Thus, we still need to know how to eliminate the buildup of stress in the body to minimize the impact of stressors we cannot eliminate. Dr. Herbert Benson has described a phenomenon called the *relaxation response* which is the opposite of the stress response. In his words,

> *Each of us possesses a natural and innate mechanism against overstress, which allows us to turn off harmful bodily effects, to counter the effects of the fight-or-flight response. This response against overstress brings on bodily changes that decrease heart rate, lower metabolism, decrease the rate of breathing, and bring the body back into what is probably a healthier balance.*

We have all experienced the pleasure of deep relaxation. Sometimes, it seems to come upon us us spontaneously: everything is going our way, the weather is beautiful, life is making few demands on us, and for a short time we feel like we don't have a care in the world.

It is possible to take active steps to bring about this state of relaxation. There are three basic avenues that we can take:

1. AWARENESS AND REGULATION OF BREATHING

2. MUSCLE RELAXATION

3. QUIETING THE MIND

Each can reduce the stress response we experience. Some, such as breathing exercises, can be utilized quickly and quietly under almost any circumstances, while others may require the proper environment. On the following pages, each of these avenues will be described in detail and exercises will be provided for putting them into practice.

Awareness and Regulation of Breathing

This is the easiest and most direct avenue to stress reduction. When we are tense or upset our breathing becomes shallow and irregular, and our heart rate tends to accelerate. When we are relaxed our breathing deepens and our heart rate decelerates. By learning to slow our breathing and to take deeper, more refreshing breaths, we can actually trigger the relaxation response. Many easily learned techniques make it possible to become more aware of our breathing and to gain control over it in ways which reduce stress.

Practice—Breathing Exercise

Instructions:

To become aware of your breathing, first, notice the difference between *breathing in* and *breathing out*. Notice the full cycle:

- INHALE: breathe in slowly and completely, filling your lungs to capacity. Notice the point when you pause before beginning to let your breath out.

- EXHALE: let your breath out completely. Now notice the moment when you have exhaled completely, before you begin another breath cycle.

Take deep breaths. Test this by putting your hand on your abdomen, just below the rib cage. Take a deep breath. As you inhale, watch your hand. Does it move in and out as your breath? It should. If it doesn't, you are breathing through your upper chest, which results in short, shallow breaths.

Notice whether you breathe through your nose or your mouth. Do you exhale completely before starting a new breath? Now put all of these parts together. Inhale through your nose. Pause for a moment and slowly allow the air to completely leave your lungs by way of your mouth. Once again pause for a moment before you start another breath cycle.

Once you become more aware of your breathing, you can use it as a tool to bring about relaxation.

EXERCISE—Reminding Ourselves to Breathe:
Programming ourselves to pay greater attention to our breathing results in increased alertness, better focus on tasks at hand, and reduced stress response.

six or eight times. Pay attention to each phase of the cycle. Also try to notice the sensations which accompany each phase of the breath cycle.

- Take a breathing break prior to starting a new activity—before making a difficult phone call, before a conference with your boss, before coming home and starting an evening with your lover or roommate.

- Take a breathing break after a stressful event. This is a good way to unwind from a tense conversation or upon hearing important news—good or bad.

EXERCISE—Rhythmic Breathing:

Once you are able to be aware of the breath cycle (inhaling, retaining, exhaling) you can enhance your relaxation by a short period of controlled rhythmic breathing. You may wish to start out limiting this exercise to six breath cycles and then returning to your regular breathing pattern.

The idea is to start with a comfortable, full inhalation. Hold your breath to a count of four, then exhale completely. The exhalation should take about twice as long as the inhalation. Pause for a moment, then repeat the breath cycle. Note your bodily sensations throughout the exercise, paying special attention to your sensations during the exhalation and final pause.

This form of patterned breathing can be used almost anywhere, at any time. It can help us calm down in a moment of stress and reduce tension. Many people use it to prepare for an important moment, such as giving a speech or facing a difficult situation. Some people claim it helps them relax and fall asleep easier when used in bed at night.

Muscle Relaxation

A second way to induce the relaxation response is through techniques of muscle relaxation. Muscles tense when we are nervous or under stress. Over time, the muscles begin to tighten up out of habit and continue to hold taut instead of returning to their normal relaxed state. This uncomfortable state of muscle tension can have serious consequences, including headaches, body aches and pains, and high blood pressure. When such responses become habitual, it becomes very difficult for the body to truly relax and release inner tension. *"Once an uptight bitch, always an uptight bitch,"* as they say.

This form of tension affects all of us at one time or another. To test for it yourself, feel the muscles in your body during an intense moment of stress. Neck, back, and shoulder muscles are the first to tighten up, but many other muscle groups are quick to follow.

There are several ways to overcome muscular tension, including stretching, exercise, and massage. If these are done on a regular basis, our muscles develop tone and resilience to the buildup of tension. When muscular tension is relieved through such techniques, stress is reduced.

Muscle tension should not be confused with muscle strength. In fact, muscles which are not used can lose their ability to hold us up properly, which can lead to backaches and disc problems.

Practice—Muscle Relaxation

MASSAGE

One of the nicest ways to combat muscular tension is very direct—massage. Although self-massage can have some effect, it is incomplete and awkward, so it is best to have someone else give our muscles a slow, careful kneading. Massage is safe; it brings us into physical contact with other people and it helps reduce stress. Rumor has it that it can sometimes even be erotic.

VARIATION 1—Get a massage from a friend:

Do a massage swap—*"I'll rub your back, if you'll rub mine."* Pick up a book on massage or take a massage class. Be sure to give both persons enough time to really relax. This may take half an hour, an hour, or more. People with experience at this recommend doing one person per day and reciprocating a day or so later. This allows both people time to rest in between and fully enjoy the massage.

VARIATION 2—Treat yourself to a massage from a professional masseur:

Paying the cost of a good masseur is well worthwhile. Look for someone properly trained, who has a sensitive, caring touch, and who relates to you as a person. Many capable masseurs and masseuses who are sensitive to gay clientele advertise in gay publications. Some advertisements, of course, are thinly disguised offers of sexual services. While sex can reduce stress, a competent professional massage is more effective. The ads usually contain some hint of what's really being sold. Physicians, therapists, and some community service organizations can often refer you to qualified masseurs.

When getting a massage, the surroundings also contribute to the experience. Clean, comfortable, aesthetically pleasing surroundings help, and some people like the added effect of a pleasant musical background. The right blend of elements can enhance the experience and help you reach a blissful, altered state of deep relaxation.

PROGRESSIVE MUSCLE RELAXATION

Relief from stress can be achieved through awareness of the sites of muscle tension and systematic relaxation of muscle groups. Numerous instructional tapes are available which can skillfully guide you through this process. Most people find they can reach a deeper state of relaxation following a skillful guide than on their own.

The following exercises will introduce you to this type of exercise, but are not a substitute for a good tape. You may wish to try out the technique before purchasing a tape. If you have a tape recorder, you may wish to read the following instructions onto a tape and play it back to yourself. This will make it easier to concentrate on the process without having to read the text.

EXERCISE #1—The Tense-and-Relax Method (requires about 15 minutes):

Sit in a straight back chair in a quiet, comfortable place. You will work through all the major muscle groups, one at a time. For each, you will complete a three step cycle: (1) fully tense the muscle and hold it for a count of five; (2) release the tension as quickly and completely as possible; (3) pause for a moment to notice the difference between the tension and relaxation. The exercise should be completed at a leisurely pace. Use the following sequence:

1. START WITH YOUR FISTS. Clench your fists—tighter—hold for a count of five while noticing the tension—RELAX and experience the relaxation. Repeat.

2. BICEPS. Bend your elbows and tighten your biceps—tighter—hold for a count of five while noticing the tension—RELAX and experience the relaxation. Repeat.

3. FACIAL MUSCLES. Close your eyes tightly. Imagine all the features of your face pushing in toward your nose. Tighten your jaw. Feel your tongue push against the roof of your mouth. Exaggerate that expression—hold for a count of five while noticing the tension—RELAX—experience the relaxation. Repeat.

4. NECK AND SHOULDERS. Imagine a force pulling backward on your forehead trying to pull your head back, while a counterforce is pulling equally on the back of your head trying to pull your head forward—feel the tension—now add to the tension by pulling your shoulders up toward your ears—hold for a count of five while noticing the tension—RELAX—experience the relaxation. Repeat.

5. Stop for a moment and take several deep, relaxed breaths. Notice the relaxation which has already come about. Compare the muscle groups which you have worked with so far to those which you have not.

6. STOMACH. Tighten your stomach muscles—hold for a count of five while noticing the tension—RELAX—experience the relaxation. Repeat.

7. LEGS AND CALVES. One leg at a time—extend your leg straight out from the chair—pull your toes toward you causing tension in the back of your leg—extend the tension by pressing outward with your heel—hold for a count of five while noticing the tension—RELAX—experience the relaxation. Repeat with other leg.

8. Once again take several complete breaths. Notice each of the muscle groups you have worked with. Allow yourself to experience the sensation of relaxation.

EXERCISE #2—Passive Progressive Relaxation:

This is similar to the previous exercise except that instead of tensing the muscle groups for a count of five, you merely focus on each area and give yourself the command to relax. Precede the exercise by a few minutes of breathing exercises. Start with your feet and work your way up the body telling yourself to relax. Pause after every command and experience the sensation of relaxation. Go slowly and be as explicit as you can about which muscle group you are asking to relax. Follow the sequence below.

1. Feet
2. Ankles
3. Calves
4. Shins
5. Knees
6. Thighs
7. Buttocks
8. Genitals
9. Stomach
10. Lower back
11. Spinal chord
12. Chest
13. Throat
14. Neck
15. Arms
16. Hands
17. Fingers
18. Forehead
19. Scalp
20. Eyes
21. Jaws
22. Tongue

Quieting the Mind

The mind is central to the creation of both stress and relaxation. For some, the mind is the serene center of our being, a place of peace, contentment, and warm colors. For others, possibly most of us, it seems more like a hornet's nest in a traffic jam. A constantly active mind, though encouraged and prized in our western culture, results in stress for many people. Unfortunately, simply telling the voices in our mind to *"shut up"* doesn't solve the problem. Other mental states are possible which do not produce stress and can actually reduce it. Techniques such as meditation and visualization which access these other states are often valued by Eastern cultures and can be learned by almost anyone.

Meditation is an ancient process for directing one's attention inward. For some, meditation has been a religious practice used to focus one's attention upon God. Recently, researchers have studied the physiological effect of meditative practices and have found significant benefits for eliciting the relaxation response.

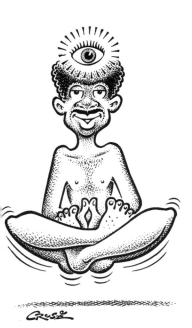

One researcher, Herbert Benson, describes four elements of meditation: a quiet environment, a mental device which provides an object to concentrate upon, a passive attitude, and a comfortable position. Of the four elements, the passive attitude appears to be the most important for triggering the relaxation response. Having a passive attitude means not focusing on any particular thoughts, images, or feelings, but letting them all pass freely through the consciousness. Furthermore, it requires avoiding judgment or evaluation of what is occurring. (The mental device, sometimes called a *gimmick*, and the passive attitude are also highly valued among practitioners of "meditation for moola." In this approach, eager students aspire to the relaxation response by relieving themselves of large sums of cash and pondering their devotion to nearly-naked gurus.)

The fundamentals of meditation can be learned easily and inexpensively. An element common to the many variations and models of meditation is an essential requirement for practice. Our minds are in the habit of active, not passive involvement, and this tendency must be overcome. With practice, meditation is said to provide deeper and more subtle benefits—both psychologically and physically. Taking a simple class or seminar is often the best way to learn these techniques—lifetime commitment to gurus is not required.

Visualization is another technique which can be used to quiet the mind. It uses positive suggestion through visual imagery to change a mental and/or physiological state. By focusing attention on a visual mental image, we can direct our attention from active thoughts. It is believed that when we create a mental picture, our bodies can actually respond to the visualization as if it were a real experience. This technique has been used as an important component in many aspects of health management, including healing, prevention, and health promotion. Although it is still unclear exactly how a mental image can affect a physiological process, research has shown that visualization can change our bodies' functioning.

Some researchers and health experts have used visualization in fighting various diseases which affect the immune system, such as cancer. Carl and Stephanie Simonton are leading proponents of this approach. Although there is still debate about the effectiveness of this approach, it is clear that visualization is an effective tool to elicit the relaxation response. When integrated into a comprehensive treatment strategy, this approach can add substantially to the psychological arsenal which can be brought to bear in combating illness.

Visualization can also assist us in reaching our goals. What we can imagine, we can accomplish. Conversely, what we cannot imagine, we cannot accomplish. Accomplishing goals takes hard work and dedication, but our dreams have a powerful influence on directing us. This can work in the reverse as well: our negative expectations also have a way of coming true.

Practice—Quieting the Mind

Start with the simple exercises below. After you master the basics, you may wish to explore more advanced techniques by further reading, use of instructional tapes, or taking instruction from a qualified teacher or therapist.

EXERCISE—Basic Meditation:

This meditative technique was developed by H. Benson and colleagues at Beth Israel Hospital and described in *The Relaxation Response* (Avon, 1975).

1. Sit quietly in a comfortable position and close your eyes.

2. Deeply relax your muscles, beginning at your feet and progressing up to your face. Keep them relaxed.

3. If possible, breathe through your nose and become aware of your breathing. Each time you breathe out (exhale), say the word "ONE" silently to yourself.

4. Maintain a passive attitude. Ignore distracting thoughts if they occur by simply concentrating on repeating step 3 above. Such distractions are common, especially when first learning how to meditate.

5. Continue for ten to twenty minutes. You may open your eyes to check the time, but do not use an alarm. When you finish, sit quietly for several minutes, at first with your eyes closed and later with your eyes opened. Do not stand up for a few minutes.

6. Avoid judging whether you've achieved a state of deep relaxation—it will come with practice. Maintain a passive attitude and permit relaxation to occur at its own pace. Practice the technique once or twice daily, but not within two hours after any meal, since the digestive processes seem to interfere with the relaxation response.

EXERCISE—Visualization:

You might wish to tape these instructions and play them back to yourself. The idea here is to first enter into a relaxed state and then add visual imagery to help deepen the relaxation.

1. Find a comfortable position—either sitting or lying down.

2. Begin with a series of breathing exercise such as those described previously.

3. As your mind calms and distractions fade away, you can focus on the various parts of your body. Give them a gentle command to relax.

4. Now picture yourself on a slow-moving escalator. Hold on to the side and slowly drift down. As you ride the escalator down, count backwards from five to one. With each count, you will become more relaxed.

5. When you finally come to the end of your escalator ride, imagine that you find yourself in your favorite outdoors place on a warm, calm, and peaceful day. Pause for a moment to notice this wonderful spot. Observe the beauty of the sky. Feel the warmth of the sun on your skin. Feel your feet on the ground under you. Smell the fresh aroma in the air. Picture yourself gently letting yourself go, sinking to the ground, letting all of the tensions in your body melt away. Continue to breathe effortlessly. With each breath you become more relaxed, more at peace. As you look up, notice beautiful billowy clouds gently passing above. Any thoughts which come to your mind, gently place them on these slow moving clouds and let them be carried away. You can stay in this perfectly safe, peaceful place as long as you wish.

6. When it's time to return, simply imagine yourself rising to your feet. Slowly walk over to the escalator and allow it to return you to the room. As you are slowly ascending, count once again—this time from one to five. On the count of three, remind yourself that when you return, to carry back the wonderful sense of relaxation, the peace of mind, and the image of yourself relaxed and happy.

EXERCISE—Visualize Health:

This visualization can be added to the previous one to promote optimal integration and functioning of the organs within our bodies. Follow the same instructions as above and start this visualization instead of #6.

1. As you sit, perfectly relaxed watching the billowy clouds pass above, imagine looking into your body. Notice the blood vessels carrying life-giving blood by way of your heart and throughout your body. Imagine with each breath your lungs filling with air; sending oxygen out through your blood. With every beat of your heart this miraculous transporting of blood and oxygen is supplying your body with the essentials of life. Spend a few minutes picturing in your mind this image. As you do this, allow your breathing to become slow and steady. See if you can hear and feel your heartbeat.

2. Now imagine within the blood, white blood cells which are the soldiers of our immune system. Imagine these cells healthy and strong. Like an army they patrol your system searching for enemy agents which do not belong. Now imagine an enemy virus. An alarm goes off and a swarm of white blood cells surrounds and destroys the outnumbered virus. The white blood cells carry the dead virus away. Now return your image to a squad of healthy white blood cells patrolling your bloodstream, keeping you healthy.

3. When you have completed your image of combating foreign agents in your body, return your attention to the larger system of heart, lungs, and blood vessels. Once again focus on your breathing and your heart beating.

4. Now, as if you are a cameraman, pull your focus back until you see yourself from the outside. Imagine yourself healthy and strong. You have plenty of energy and your outlook is cheerful and hopeful. You feel confident of your own abilities and feel good about yourself. You feel comfortable with being gay and have a loving appreciation for other people.

5. Carrying this positive attitude with you, you may return to the room by locating the escalator which brought you to this healing place. Remember to count to five on your way up and to return slowly.

Action Plan—Stress Reduction

Instructions:

After you've familiarized yourself with at least three of the techniques described in the previous pages, list below those which you have practiced and intend to use in your overall stress management effort. Briefly describe what you hope to get out of it and how you plan to integrate it into your regular activities, or under what circumstances you will use it.

Technique: _____

WHY I will use it: _____

_____

WHEN I will use it: _____

_____

Technique: _____

WHY I will use it: _____

_____

WHEN I will use it: _____

_____

Technique: _____

WHY I will use it: _____

_____

WHEN I will use it: _____

_____

**STEP 4:
IMPLEMENTING THE
PLAN**

Many experts feel that stress reduction hinges on the seemingly simple ability to learn to relax. The various techniques are only tools to help accomplish this. The techniques you read about here can be supplemented by others which are widely available. Good alternatives include the various schools of meditation, chanting, relaxation tapes, and numerous stress management seminars and programs. In considering the options, we need to be good consumers, protecting ourselves from overly aggressive commercial interests. There are many, many effective techniques and there is no need to become dogmatically dependent on one approach versus another.

Stress reduction skills can be learned by anyone, but they require practice and patience to develop. One advantage of formalized training is that it provides a motivational environment which supports practicing the techniques which have been learned. This goes awry only when the system digs too deeply into our pockets or closes us off from other helpful experiences.

The effectiveness of any stress reduction strategy is mostly dependent on practice and methodical application of the techniques—not on the beliefs of the guru behind them. For many people, a comforting weekend at the beach can have profound benefits, with or without any special techniques.

Stress prevention and stress reduction should be a part of almost everyone's overall health strategy. All of us are affected by the AIDS crisis, and the extra stress provided is the last thing we need. How often we use the stress reduction exercises should vary depending upon the degrees of stress we are experiencing. For example, under extremely stressful circumstances, breathing exercises might be done several times a day and adapted to the place in which we do them, such as the workplace.

To supplement such on-the-spot techniques, we might seek the long-lasting effects achieved by a daily practice of meditation or deep relaxation. When seeking these benefits, you need to set aside at least twenty minutes per setting, at least once a day. Twice a day is even better. The best times for practicing these techniques are:

- when first rising

- around 3:00 p.m. (a natural break to refuel your energies)

- in the evening.

STRESS REDUCTION routines can even help eliminate chronic stress which has built up over time. The breathing exercises provide a good antidote for moments of acute stress since they can be practiced at work before a stressful meeting, interview, or anxiety-provoking situation. You'll find them useful not only for reducing the level of stress, but also for putting you at your best, relaxed and confident as you undertake the tasks before you.

A final important aspect of managing stress is to be sure to take special care of yourself before and after stressful situations. One way to do this is to use the process of visualization. You can do this by utilizing your mind's eye to imagine yourself unstressed, feeling relaxed, confident, content and having a sense of well-being.

A Health Perspective

Drug Use and the Gay Community

Use, Abuse, and Dependency

The Track Record of Individual Drugs

CHAPTER

4

SUBSTANCE USE AND ABUSE

INTRODUCTION

It is no secret that many gay men have had an ongoing affair with consciousness-altering substances. Gay people played center stage in the "age of Aquarius" in the 60's and virtually created the neon "disco, dancing, and drugs" scene of the 70's so widely emulated in today's trendy straight clubs. Using illicit drugs was but another small step for those who had already crossed the lines of sexual conformity.

Long before crack, cheap cocaine, and animal tranquilizers masquerading as aphrodisiacs, there was a time when the environment supported the notion of better living through chemistry. Psychiatrists experimented in earnest with the journeys afforded by LSD and MDA, artists and everyday people explored new colors of life filtered through the smoke of a burning plant. Many gay people seemed especially drawn to the lure of chemical change. Some felt it brought new awakenings, new awareness of inner feelings, and a capacity for uninhibited passion. More than a few lasting gay unions began in the warm haze of chemically inspired lust. For some, however, drugs became the only way to feel anything at all.

As a group, we've all had to carry heavy emotional baggage and some turned to drugs and alcohol hoping to ease the burden. Yet, sooner or later, most users learned there was a dark side to drugs. Coming down often proved more painful than never going up. Elation and passion weren't far removed from confusion and terror. Dreamy visions gave way to the harsh glare of crystal and needles. For every relationship forged in the heat of chemistry, dozens more were shattered in the sobering light of dawn.

As in most human endeavors, our greatest failing was not knowing when to quit, or not realizing until it was too late that we couldn't if we wanted to. For some, drugs and alcohol led to despair and addiction. Whatever weaknesses we harbored came boiling to the surface, often with a power we never imagined.

Finding a responsible path through this mix of enticement, faded dreams, and the harsh realities of AIDS is the aim of this chapter.

A HEALTH PERSPECTIVE

There's little argument these days that substance DEPENDENCY and ABUSE are deadly propositions, especially in light of the threat of AIDS. Yet substance USE has long been a part of our gay culture and it clearly hasn't destroyed everyone who made it so. Finding the lines between dependency, abuse, and use is the personal challenge we must face if we choose to indulge at all.

For starters, we need a common definition. When the words *"substance"* or *"drug"* are used in this text, they may refer to any and all of the following:

ALCOHOL—including beer, wine, and hard liquors;

COMMON STREET CHEMICALS—such as speed (crystal), downers, acid, MDA, angel dust, cocaine, crack, freebase cocaine, Ecstasy, and other "designer" concoctions;

PRESCRIPTION DRUGS—such as sleeping pills, diet pills, pain pills, tranquilizers;

PSYCHOACTIVE PLANTS—such as tobacco, marijuana, and mushrooms.

Limiting discussion of substance abuse on the basis of legal classifications is one of the great hypocrisies of our era. Substances responsible for the greatest social and personal consequences—alcohol and tobacco—are often given a free ride because society is still so strongly dependent on them. Legal consequences, while of great personal importance, are not our concern here. Since homosexual behavior itself remains illegal in many states, this book obviously cannot confine its discourse within existing legal boundaries. Possession or use of illegal drugs, however, includes the potential for arrest, and each user must determine how the expected benefits stack up against the risks.

Finally, conventional "moral" considerations are also beyond the scope of this discussion. Gay people have always had to cut their own path through the restrictions imposed by conventional morality.

Since the goal of this book is to assist in the battle against AIDS—not to influence or conform to legal or social practices—all substances will be examined equitably from the perspective of health. No permission to break the law or contradict one's own standards of morality, however, should in any way be inferred.

Physical Consequences of Drug Use

Approximately one in ten Americans is a problem drinker or is chemically dependent at some point in their life. Proceeding from the perspective of health, a number of undeniable facts must be faced.

- Drugs (including alcohol) are a factor in a majority of automobile fatalities, suicides, homicides and other violent crimes.

- The psychological complications of drug abuse are known to damage careers, personal relationships, and mental health.

- Numerous medical conditions are directly linked to the use and abuse of drugs (these account for more than 20% of all hospital admissions in the United States):

    BRAIN AND NERVOUS SYSTEM, signs and symptoms:
    - Fatigue
    - Overdose
    - Seizures
    - Depression
    - Reduced sex drive
    - Ataxia (unsteady gait)
    - Peripheral neuropathy (numbness, tingling in arms or legs)
    - Temporary nerve palsies
    - Impaired memory, judgment and concentration
    - Confabulation (storytelling to fill gaps in memory)

DIGESTIVE SYSTEM, signs and symptoms:
- Hepatitis, jaundice, ascites (loss of fluid into the abdomen)
- Peripheral edema (swelling of hands and feet)
- Bruising
- Malnutrition
- Weight gain or loss
- Gastric pain, gas, distension
- Nausea and vomiting
- Inflammation or ulcers of the mouth, throat, esophagus, stomach, pancreas, small or large intestines
- Diarrhea or constipation
- Stomach or abdominal cramps

RESPIRATORY SYSTEM, signs and symptoms:
- Shortness of breath
- Diminished cough reflex
- Difficulty coughing up fluids or mucus
- Increased respiratory infections/pneumonia

CARDIOVASCULAR SYSTEM, signs and symptoms:
- Elevated or irregular heart rate
- Hypertension (high blood pressure)
- Enlarged heart
- Endocarditis (inflammation of the heart lining)
- Decreased exercise tolerance and fatigue
- Transient chest pain
- Peripheral edema (swelling of hands and feet)

IMMUNE SYSTEM, signs and symptoms:
- Increased incidence and prolonged duration of infection
- Impaired ability to fight infection
- Increased incidence of cancer
- Transmission of hepatitis and AIDS (through shared hypodermic needles)
- High correlation between use of "poppers" and development of Kaposi's sarcoma

Four variables affect the severity of drug-related health problems:

(1) THE CHEMISTRY AND PHYSICAL EFFECTS of the particular drug or combination of drugs used: different drugs produce very different results, straining and interacting with various body systems and processes.

(2) THE AMOUNT of the drug(s) used: this includes cumulative totals as well as the total amount taken at any one time.

(3) THE FREQUENCY of drug use.

(4) THE UNDERLYING HEALTH of the individual, including genetic vulnerability: studies of the children of alcoholic parents strongly imply a genetic link in alcoholism; research suggests that alcoholics' bodies metabolize alcohol differently than non-alcoholics.

Almost everyone with any kind of a drug problem tends to underestimate the severity of one or more of these variables.

Viewed from the perspective of health, it would be hard to argue that any level of repeated drug use is inconsequential. Likewise, it is hard to argue that all drug use results in serious harm. Thus, it is unrealistic to assume that everyone needs to or will "just say no."

Prohibition, severe criminal penalties, exaggerated drug horror stories, and even such absurdities as poisoning drugs with toxic agents have all failed to eliminate or even diminish public consumption. Obviously, chemically altered consciousness has a strong and continuing appeal to a large percentage of the population.

Drugs and AIDS

Whatever the arguments are about drug use in general, they hold special concern for people at risk or already infected by the AIDS virus. The role of drugs as a complicating factor in AIDS has long been established. Two key questions arise:

What is the total health impact of drug use, both for those who are ill with AIDS or ARC and for those who are at risk?

What special role, if any, do drugs play in the risk of developing AIDS and ARC?

The frequency of drug use often misleads researchers in developing an early understanding of the illness. Early studies noted two lifestyle characteristics of early AIDS patients: (1) a high degree of gay sexual activity and (2) a history of drug use. For some time, it was suspected that drug abuse might well be a co-factor in the development of the disease. Later studies reached an altered conclusion.

While many early patients did have drug experience and were very active sexually, people with no history of drug use were also found to be at risk. Drug use and a high degree of sexual activity were closely linked for many people, leading at least to increased risk of exposure. This was especially true if needles were involved. But the notion of a

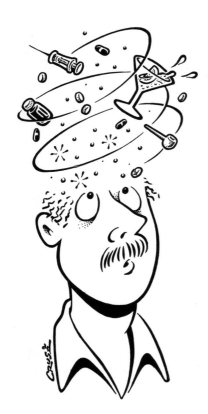

strong cause and effect link between AIDS and the effects of drug use (other than shared needles) was not proven by research.

The relationship between AIDS and drug use, however, is significant. A few facts which highlight this connection:

FACT: More than twenty-five percent of people with AIDS or AIDS-related conditions admit to drug or alcohol problems.

FACT: IV drug use (sharing needles) has been identified as a major means of transmission of the AIDS virus.

FACT: Some drugs have a direct suppressive effect on the immune system which may increase both the risk and severity of infection by the AIDS virus.

FACT: Many drugs, including alcohol, interfere with many types of treatment for AIDS.

FACT: Drugs alter judgment, feelings, and perceptions—this is often the reason for using them. Altered judgment makes many people more prone to engage in high-risk sexual activities, interferes with diet and health routines, and can easily lead people to push themselves beyond their limits.

FACT: Drug use causes stress rather than helping cope with it. Excessive stress directly harms the functioning of the immune system.

On the whole, this is not a pretty picture. Yet not everyone who uses drugs has a bad experience. While the *"just say no"* crowd doesn't like to hear it, some people claim to be able to integrate a degree of drug use into their lives with little apparent short-term harm. In some instances, an arguable case can be made that such drug use provides a degree of short term benefits. Some of this falls into the *"hey, I can handle it"* category of denial, but, in fact, occasional drug use seems harmless for some people. This is unlikely to be true, however, for at least three categories of people:

- people who may be genetically predisposed to dependency, such as the children of alcoholic parents;

- people who seem inclined toward self-destructive behavior;

- people whose immune system is weakened by the AIDS virus.

It should be evident that if the drug experience were as black and white as the moralists claim, it would have faded from human practice long ago. It hasn't, and thus the dilemma and challenge we face.

Drug Use and the Gay Community

Our community's experience with drugs has not been all flower power, sexual passion, and psychedelic colors. The rate of alcoholism and chemical dependency in the gay and lesbian communities is three times that of the general population. It is thus a major contributing factor of death in our community.

Gay people are not the first or only minority group with a disproportionate number of drug abusers. Yet, critics often cite this as evidence of moral weakness in our community. Others see it as a response to the oppression and discrimination we suffer. A true picture is broader than either of these views. Several factors probably contribute to the abuse of alcohol and drugs in our community:

• the stress of being gay in a non-gay world;

• the pressures of internalized homophobia which bear upon our sexual activities;

• the importance of the bar as our traditional meeting place;

• our inherent status of being "outside the law."

Most of us have a past, present, and future which includes some degree of oppression. Growing up gay hasn't been easy for any of us and living in a decidedly non-gay world is eased only somewhat by becoming part of a community. Many have sought solace from a bottle, pill, or syringe.

Many gay social activities and traditions also encourage the use of drugs. Bars have long been our foremost meeting place, one of the few environments in which we can be entirely "out," where we need no pretensions of heterosexuality. Drinking, not socializing, is what keeps bars in business. Likewise, the intensity of our dance clubs and the dark intrigue of leather and "scene" clubs have been fueled by alcohol, amyl, crystal, coke, downers, and psychedelics. Growing up in this environment, we've found plenty of camaraderie in the use of drugs and little encouragement for sobriety. In some instances, even physicians who are part of our community have been swept along by the beat, winking at our use of "recreational drugs." Before AIDS, we heard few negative messages about drugs from each other.

Today, however, there are strong voices in our community calling out for reconsideration of our drug usage, for a more sober future.

Drugs and sex have become closely associated for many of us. Some say their sexual activities are always accompanied by drugs—and have been for years. The highest highs, most intense orgasms, and greatest passions are sometimes linked with the drug of choice. Some say they just aren't able to let go, to reach out, to get loose—or hard—without chemical inducement. At the very least, it becomes a powerful habit; once established, it's difficult to imagine it any other way.

How did it come to this? Is it, as the moralists believe, proof of how deviant our sexuality really is? Hardly (if you'll pardon the pun).

Sex presents a dilemma for many gay people (perhaps for straight people too). It is perhaps the strongest expression of what makes us different, yet, at the same time, it forces us to confront our difference and all the homophobia pounded into us since childhood. While sexual guilt is common throughout American society, gay people must face a special chorus of taboos whenever the lights dim. For many, a drug-induced state has been the only way to get past the hangups and around to the passion. This is most vivid when we cross the line for the first time and "come out." Thereafter, from friends, lovers, and seducers alike, we learn repeatedly that drugs and alcohol make it all seem so much easier.

USE, ABUSE, AND DEPENDENCY

For better of worse, the social or "recreational" use of drugs is deeply ingrained in our community. For the majority of people, this has created few apparent problems. For some, none at all—especially those who shun drugs and alcohol altogether. Although our attitude toward drugs is already being reevaluated in light of AIDS, it's unrealistic to think that all drug use will simply disappear. For practical purposes, there are at least three categories which describe the drug and alcohol experience:

    1. DEPENDENCY

    2. ABUSE

    3. USE

Any of the three categories may include elements of another. A person can move in both directions between USE and ABUSE and either can lead to DEPENDENCY. But there is only a one-way street to DEPENDENCY—once there, a person cannot go back to being a USER or ABUSER. Each category describes a distinct level of involvement with drugs, a distinct level of consequences.

Dependency

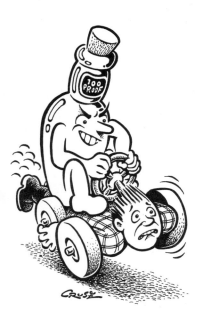

Some people seem to cross an invisible line and lose control of their alcohol or drug use. At this point, one no longer needs a "reason" to drink or use drugs. Each of us needs to know where that line is, and on what side of it we stand. Although the reasons why a person develops drug DEPENDENCY are not fully understood, evidence suggests that both genetics and early childhood experiences may play a role. People who develop DEPENDENCY to one drug often become dependent on others as well. The phenomenon, known as cross-dependence, is common with alcohol and other "downers." Drug DEPENDENCY is considered to be a disease—not a moral condition—a progressive illness requiring treatment. It can only be contained by complete abstinence, typically from all drugs, not just the source of the DEPENDENCY.

Recognizing the early stages of drug DEPENDENCY, including alcoholism, is elusive, especially when we don't want to see it. Few find it difficult to spot full-scale DEPENDENCY among the homeless on the "skid rows" of every major town. And each of us can pick it out in one or another of our acquaintances:

- the braying, perpetual drunk—on the street, in the bar, on the dance floor, even at work;

- the guy who's always face down in the punch bowl at parties;

- the hyperactive sister blowing coke or speed up her nose at 8 in the morning;

- that one over there, the one who's into needles;

- the ex-roommate, friend, or lover whose drinking or drugging ruined our relationship.

Are these the drug addicts and alcoholics in your life? Maybe, maybe not. Drug dependency and alcoholism can't always be spotted, especially in ourselves. No aspect of life is more prone to denial, whether it's about ourselves, our friends, or our lovers. Dependency comes in all shapes, sizes, and forms.

How effectively do we recognize these others?

- the banker, lawyer, doctor, guy with a solid job, a house, nice car—and a private habit;

- the friend we go out with to cut loose for an evening—the one who always stays out just a little longer than we do;

- the sex buddy who's always taken us just a little higher, while always staying in control—every time we get it on;

- the guy in the mirror, whose life seems to be working okay—who can stop anytime he wants.

It's difficult to look at a successful person and see DEPENDENCY beneath the facade. Chemical dependency provides rich opportunities for denial, both for the dependent and for those who care about him. For example, in the middle stages of alcoholism, it is common for alcoholics to integrate their dependency into what looks like a normal life. The guy who "holds his liquor" well at parties can be just as much an alcoholic as the obvious drunk.

When does USE or ABUSE become DEPENDENCY? In the upcoming "Step One" of this chapter, you'll have a chance to ask yourself a few questions to help assess this personally. In general, recovering addicts report a few common indicators. When:

- the drug of choice becomes the most important aspect of life (a main consideration in finances, shopping, and use of free time);

- we don't leave home without it (the drug of choice);

- anxiety quickly builds if the supply runs out;

- we don't socialize without it;

- we find that most people we associate with are using the same substance or support our use of it;

- we're content to spend time alone with our favorite drug;

- we can't relax without it;

- we hear ourselves arguing that none of these points are true, yet a doubting voice inside says they are;

DEPENDENCY doesn't always mean taking or using the drug every day. While this is one common model of dependency, it isn't the only one. Some addicts go for days without drinking or using a drug, then go on a "binge." This model provides an excellent opportunity for rationalization and denial. Yet the "binging" addict is no less dependent than the "everyday" addict. Some recovering addicts report that they created or used a variety of life events—disappointments, setbacks, failed romances—as an excuse to justify going on the next binge. For some, the binge was the objective all along, not a response to problems in their lives.

Sometimes, people recognize their own DEPENDENCY only when they "hit bottom," a phrase whose meaning is totally personal and subjective. The most fortunate addicts are those who acknowledge their problem before that "bottom" is too extreme. Confronting dependency, whether to street drugs, alcohol, or prescription drugs, is one of the greatest challenges an individual can undertake. The factors which make a person an addict, whatever they are, never go away. There can never be occasional or "recreational" use of a substance for an addict. The only solution is total and lasting abstinence.

Which substances are capable of producing dependency? Although some drugs such as alcohol and heroin are singled out for their strong physical powers of addiction, almost any drug is capable of producing the phenomenon. Many experts no longer distinguish between "physically" and "psychologically" addictive substances. Both destroy the lives and hopes of the addict.

If dependency only affected the person with the problem, it would be serious enough. Unfortunately, the harm done extends in a wide circle around the addict. Close friends and lovers, out of loyalty and concern, rarely escape the suffering. Often, they come to play a part in the pattern of destruction which emerges. The damage takes many forms for the friends, lovers, and family. Financial drain, physical abuse and stress, emotional trauma and guilt, and social isolation or embarrassment are just a few of the most common results.

Dependency, like other serious illnesses, cannot be conquered alone. Professional help and peer group assistance is the required therapy. If you suspect that you or someone you love has a drug dependency, get help from the many resources which are available. People who expect to kick their habits alone are simply engaging in another level of denial. Throughout the U.S., there is a growing body of support for gay people with drug problems. Gay AA (Alcoholics Anonymous) and NA (Narcotics Anonymous) groups are available in most cities and have a great deal of experience in helping, even for people who once thought they could "do it alone."

When help is sought, it commonly includes help for the loved ones as well as the addict. In many instances, the loved ones cry out for help well before the addict acknowledges he has a problem. Whether help is for the addict or his loved ones, it's important to use a counselor or service which is sensitive to gay lifestyles.

Drug dependency, and alcoholism in particular, have created much individual and community turmoil. Although few plan on becoming addicted, it happens, slowly and insidiously, nonetheless. Once a problem or potential problem exists, it will almost certainly get worse without help. To get help, the addict needs to reach out and take responsibility—it can't be forced on him by others.

Dependency and AIDS   AIDS, of course, brings its own complications and connections to the world of the addict. Sharing needles is the second most common source of AIDS transmission, and probably the most reliable. While other dependencies don't always provide such a deadly direct risk, they all seriously affect the judgment, behaviors, and attention to health of the addict. Alcoholics take far too many of their calories in the form of alcohol, thus robbing their bodies of essential nutrients. Nicotine addicts—cigarette dependency—lose a little bit of life with every puff. Amphetamines rob the AIDS-infected drug dependent of his already limited resources. Many drugs directly counteract the benefits of critically needed medical treatments.

A few facts about drug dependency and AIDS are well established:

FACT: Addicts with AIDS have a considerably shorter life expectancy than AIDS patients in general.

FACT: Addicts are harder to reach with treatment efforts.

FACT: Addicts' emotional and social support systems are typically less effective.

FACT: Financial problems created by AIDS become overwhelming for addicts.

In short, an addict with AIDS is a grave danger to himself and to those around him. The first step for an addict living with AIDS must be an immediate confrontation with his dependencies.

For people with ARC or who test positive to the AIDS virus, several predictions can responsibly be made from the data on AIDS patients. Drug dependency seems very likely to increase the risk or rate of conversion to more serious forms of the disease. Those who are sick seem likely to experience a greater number of opportunistic infections. Psychologically, they are inclined, by habit, to engage in extended denial before confronting their illness.

The bottom line is quite clear. Drug dependency makes any level of AIDS infection worse than it needs to be.

A Special Case: Tobacco Dependency

Tobacco dependency—addiction to cigarettes—is perhaps the most common form of dependency. A disproportionately large percentage of the population is addicted to cigarette smoking. Despite recent trends to the contrary, it remains the most socially acceptable addiction. The medical dangers have been well known for decades and are disputed only by the Tobacco Institute.

Every smoker knows the danger and is sick of hearing about it. If this includes you, don't tune out. Continue reading if you possibly can.

The risk of AIDS demands confrontation with the rationalizations for continued use of tobacco. Research conducted since the beginning of the epidemic cries out to the smokers among us. Previously, smoking was strongly implicated in lung disease, lung and mouth cancers, heart disease, hardening of the arteries, and stomach disorders. The new research adds several new complications:

- the presence of lung infections, often associated with AIDS, enhances the cancer-causing properties of smoking;

- smoking causes several types of immune system suppression;

- smoking is strongly associated with increased occurrence and severity of lung disease in AIDS patients;

- smoking is strongly associated with slower recovery from lung illnesses, including pneumocystis pneumonia;

- smoking increases the likelihood and spread of common skin cancers (melanomas);

- smoking acts together with alcohol to produce oral cancers.

Smoking adds serious burdens for patients with AIDS or ARC, and increases the likelihood of illness for those at risk. In a recent visit to an AIDS hospital ward in San Francisco, Surgeon General Koop was confronted by a patient, cigarette in his hand, who asked for his advice. A visibly irritated Koop shouted back at the patient:

"Stop smoking! You'll feel a lot better."

The physicians, friends, and lovers of smokers share this frustration. The damage of smoking is so clear, so obvious, that it is hard to stand by without confronting it.

Those of us who have been smokers, however, know that no one but ourselves can make the change. If a smoker wants to live, wants to have his best shot at combating AIDS or ARC or preventing exposure from progressing to illness, physicians say that getting help with a smoking problem is the single most important step a person can take.

Those who have tried and failed should get help—there's plenty around. Anti-smoking clinics and seminars, counselling services, support groups, hypnotism—all have been shown to help people who want to quit. Cigarette addiction is among the most powerful; there is no shame, no weakness, in admitting that we need help to stop. Most of the effects, most of the damage, are reversible. Can cigarettes possibly be worth it?

Abuse

Not everyone who has ever had trouble with drugs or alcohol is an addict. People who demonstrate none of the characteristics of addiction sometimes become the loud drunk, the guy with the glaring eyes, or the nodding queen in the corner. In fact, few of us can pretend we haven't had a moment or two which gave our friends something to worry about. Whether addicts or not, we feel the pressures of being gay in a hostile world, and we all occasionally seek relief. Addicts or not, most of us have gotten high, even exceeded our personal limits, just because "it felt good."

In the "good old days," as we're already calling them, overindulgence was far from the exception. Yet not everyone was or became dependent. The pressures and agonies of AIDS itself have so added to our psychological burdens that it is difficult to fault ourselves or our friends for sporadic moments of madness. We live with the pallor of death around us, with the shattering loss of young, vibrant friends and lovers, with confusion and anxiety over our own futures.

Two key questions must be faced:

Where is the line between ABUSE and DEPENDENCY, and between USE and ABUSE?

What are the implications of ABUSE for those at risk and those who are already ill?

The lines between DEPENDENCY and ABUSE are drawn by the appearance or nonappearance of the characteristics of dependency discussed in the previous section.

Three factors help point out the line between ABUSE and USE: (1) the degree to which the quantity of the drug used affects a person's behavior, (2) the conditions under which the drug is used, and (3) the results of the drug use on a person's life.

On the simplest level, ABUSE of drugs may be described as any use beyond that for which the drug is intended. This model is clearest when applied to prescription drugs.

Prescription drugs are abused when taken in greater amounts or more frequently than is recommended, or for conditions other than those prescribed. For practical purposes, this means when we take the drug to get high, rather than to relieve the conditions for which it was prescribed. Using a drug like Valium™ to party rather than strictly as the doctor ordered is a fairly popular form of abuse. Gulping Percodan™ to loosen up out on the dance floor also qualifies as abuse.

ABUSE is harder to define when applied to alcohol. We are told that alcohol manufacturers do not knowingly promote drunkenness as the purpose of their products. It is this smug presumption of moderate use which allows legislators to pretend alcohol isn't a drug. Alcohol ABUSE might be described as drinking to drunkenness or until it interferes with normal life functions. By this definition, most drinkers abuse alcohol once in a while; most would admit to doing so. Society, straight and gay alike, provides plenty of support for occasional bouts of drunkenness. Sometimes, alcohol ABUSE is defined not by how much we drink, but by the circumstances. Getting a little loaded at home before going to sleep is quite different from doing so before driving a car—yet the quantity of alcohol may be the same. The difference lies in the potential results.

Since street drugs and psychoactive plants, including tobacco, seldom have valid purposes, defining their ABUSE is a highly subjective matter. From the viewpoint of law, any USE is ABUSE. In the real world, this is arguable on a substance-by-substance basis. IV drug use, regardless of the substance involved, almost always implies a commitment that always goes beyond mere USE of a drug, and almost always beyond ABUSE to DEPENDENCY.

Tobacco, a legal drug, is so strongly addictive that virtually everyone who smokes more than a few times becomes dependent. There is little distance between USE and DEPENDENCY.

Marijuana is an easier example. Many people smoke marijuana only on rare occasions and seldom think of it when it is unavailable. This can be categorized as marijuana USE. Others, however, keep a constant supply handy and perhaps smoke it at breaks while working or while driving. ABUSE and USE can be defined in much the same way they are with alcohol. If the amount (or strength) of what's smoked interferes with normal functions, it can be categorized as ABUSE. Some will argue that interference with the "normal" state is precisely why it is smoked in the first place. To determine USE or ABUSE, we need to look at the results on a person's life.

The discussion of other street drugs must also be handled on a case-by-case basis. One could argue that almost any drug could be used or abused. The labelling can be based on (1) the amount/frequency of use, (2) the degree to which use interferes with normal functions, and (3) the results. For many people, the distinction is entirely personal: USE becomes ABUSE when, after careful and honest examination, a person feels it is a problem.

Once a person acknowledges drug ABUSE in his life, he must decide what to do about it. In most instances, drugs are abused for a reason, consciously or unconsciously. To change, a person must explore those reasons, examine what he feels he is getting out of drugs, and how to get it another way. This can be done in private counselling, in groups, or, in some cases, with the help of a caring friend.

Use

Drug USE is the easiest of all categories to define, a simple on/off, yes/no consideration. If you drink, swallow, inject, smoke, or snort any of the substances classified here as drugs, you engage in drug use. As in the other categories, the significance of such use is determined by the four variables listed previously:

(1)   the chemistry and physical effects of the particular drug or combination of drugs used;

(2)   the amount of the drug(s) used;

(3)   the frequency of drug use;

(4)   the underlying health of the individual.

Each of us must assess the impact of drugs in our lives and must determine whether our behavior constitutes USE, ABUSE, or DEPENDENCY.

On first glance, we may be very inclined to categorize our behavior as drug USE. Some degree of denial is likely because honest introspection runs the risk of requiring change. We've already had to make sexual changes, perhaps giving up our favorite practices. Now, we are asked to weigh the risks and benefits of what for many is a tradition of drug use. Whether we make changes or not, we at least must examine what we do and understand the consequences.

To some extent, denial can be minimized if we avoid making value judgments about ourselves or others when we use the terms like USE, ABUSE, and DEPENDENCY. While drug DEPENDENCY is a problem, the drug DEPENDENT is not a bad person because of it. Drug USERS are not automatically better persons than drug ABUSERS. And NON-USERS aren't necessarily better than any of them. Each term simply describes a category of behavior. Deciding who's good or bad, or what's good or bad for you is a separate matter.

Use, Abuse and AIDS

Before AIDS, an arguable case could be made that some drug use was relatively harmless. After all, the government for decades has implied this is so for alcohol and tobacco. Gay people (and many others) have simply extended the list.

Problems associated with drug USE and ABUSE are amplified by the presence of AIDS in our community and our lives. Two themes referenced throughout this book recur in this context:

• *the risk of contracting or spreading the disease;*

• *our ability to fight it.*

There is little question that both are affected by the nature and severity of drug abuse. Most forms of drug abuse are frequently associated with high-risk sexual behavior. The willing sense of abandon, the level of permission we give ourselves is far greater when we are "under the influence." Drugs are commonly used to overcome inhibitions, to extend the threshold of pain, and have been deeply integrated into many people's sexual activities.

Unfortunately, AIDS demands something more of us than totally uninhibited behavior. Like it not, we need to set reasonable limits in the bedroom to protect our right to a future. While drugs may well have helped many people overcome deep-rooted sexual inhibitions, they also diminish concern for legitimate limits.

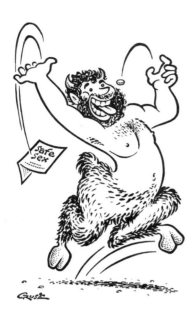

Almost everyone knows what's safe and what's not these days and few are happy about the limitations this imposes. In a sober state, rational thinking tells us what to do. Under the influence, primal urges and our dicks lead the way. In the soft haze of alcohol, the swirling sensations of psychedelics, or the glaring intensity of amphetamines, it's far too easy to forget or to knowingly let it happen, "just this one time." And one time is all it takes.

If we are not infected but risk contact with the virus, we don't know when infection might occur. If infected but not sick, we live with the risk that a dormant virus may suddenly progress to a more active disease state. If we are sick with any degree of ARC, we don't know how close we are to crossing the imaginary line to AIDS. For some, there is a gradual deterioration and plenty of warning. For many others, the change is sudden and unexpected. Having the strongest possible defenses at any of these critical moments makes obvious sense. When the stakes are so high, every possible advantage must be sought, every disadvantage blocked. There is little argument that ongoing dependencies are more damaging to our health than occasional drug abuse. Yet, under the pressures created by the AIDS virus, every event counts.

Some of the best advice can be heard from those already fallen ill, reciting the personal litany of *"if only"*:

> *"If only I had gone on the wagon when it could still help. . ."*

> *"If only I had laid off the hard drugs. . ."*

> *"If only I had never gotten into needles . . ."*

> *"If only I had saved the money I blew on coke . . ."*

> *"If only I had quit when I had the strength to care . . ."*

Each of us need only project our own "if only's" to know where to start making changes.

THE TRACK RECORD OF INDIVIDUAL DRUGS

Before examining the impact of the drug or drugs we use or abuse, it's necessary to take a broad look at what's know about them. Research is clearest when it comes to the best known drugs: alcohol, tobacco, and prescription drugs. All have been studied extensively over the last 50 years. In the case of alcohol and tobacco, the results are shocking. Had the potential for damage been known decades ago, it is likely that both drugs would be on the forbidden list. Once a drug is ingrained in society the way alcohol and tobacco are, it is extremely difficult to take them away. This argument is widely used to continue prohibitions against other drugs which, at least for the moment, appear to be less harmful.

Most drug research is lacking substance in the area of impact on the immune system. A great deal of what's known about the immune system has been learned only recently in the study of AIDS. As a result of this late start, extensive data simply isn't available on how each drug affects complex immune responses. There are, however, strong suspicions that many drugs counteract the body's efforts to protect itself. Similarly, many of the drugs discussed here are known to interact in a harmful way with many of the drugs used in the treatment of AIDS.

In the absence of conclusive data on many drugs, the only safe assumption is that they are at least not likely to help the immune system—and will probably hurt it.

Read the following table concerning the drugs previously discussed. For each drug, the most common physical effects are listed in the column labelled "Direct Effects." The next column, labelled "Indirect Effects," lists secondary effects widely believed to be associated with the drug. In the final column, known effects on interaction with AIDS treatments or recovery processes are listed. When you've finished examining the table, go on to the next exercise to further evaluate your personal situation.

And don't get bent out of shape if your favorite "recreational" high gets a bad rap. Maybe your use of the drug is so moderate, so cool, that you never bump into the gremlins lurking within. It's also possible that you haven't been a "user" long enough for the effects to occur. The damage from most drugs is long-term and cumulative. The impact of any drug use is determined by the four variables mentioned previously—not just the drug itself. But don't discount the information out of hand simply because it doesn't agree with your own experience or because you don't want to hear it.

Drug	Direct Effects	Indirect Effects	AIDS-related Effects
ALCOHOL	Liver and heart damage; stomach, intestinal, and esophagal damage; anemia; nerve and brain damage; powerful physical addiction.	Lowered inhibitions; depression; impaired perception and motor coordination; increased anxiety; diminished sensitivity to pain (allows physical harm to go unnoticed); conducive to high-risk sexual activity.	Lowers effectiveness of antibiotic and antiviral drugs; immuno-suppression; increased incidence and duration of infection; may encourage growth of oral candida (thrush); complication in treatment of brain disorders.
COCAINE (including free-base and crack)	Heart and lung damage; stroke; cardiovascular irregularities; possible physical addiction.	Distortion of judgment, values, and senses; dangerous delusions of grandeur and strength; intense anxiety, paranoia; financial strain; leads to poor judgment about highrisk sexual activity.	Likely immuno-suppression (not currently measured); increased stress; if smoked, complicates treatment of pneumonia.
DOWNERS (tranquilizers, sedatives, hypnotics, sleeping pills)	Suppression of autonomic systems, such as breathing and heartbeat (in overdose); potential for lethal overdose; possible powerful physical addiction.	Passivity, suggestibility; distortion of judgment, values, and senses; lowered sensitivity to pain; conducive to high-risk passive sexual activity; potential for psychological addiction.	Possible immuno-suppression (not currently measured); slows healing processes; potential for unknown and risky drug interactions.
HYBRIDS (MDA, Ecstasy, designer drugs)	Effects vary greatly by drug and by batch; possible liver damage; possible neural and heart damage (MDA); amphetamine-like damage; high risk of unknown, impure chemicals.	Severe alterations in perception and judgment; very conducive to high-risk sexual activity; extreme suggestibility; similar to psychedelics and amphetamines.	Unknown; very likely immuno-suppression.
MARIJUANA	Potential for lung damage with regular use.	Impaired judgment; inducement of high-risk sexual activity; potential for psychological addiction.	Possible immuno-suppression (not consistently established by current research).

Drug	Direct Effects	Indirect Effects	AIDS-related Effects
OPIATES (heroin, morphine, codeine, other pharmaceuticals)	Suppression of autonomic systems, such as breathing and heartbeat (in overdose); interference with digestive processes; high potential for severe physical addiction.	Extreme passivity, suggestibility; distortion of judgment, values, and senses; lowered sensitivity to pain; severe financial strain; very conducive to high-risk sexual activity.	Unknown.
POPPERS (amyl nitrate and nitrites)	Possible heart damage; fibrillation (compulsive, erratic heart rhythms); possible stroke and resulting brain damage.	Conducive to high-risk sexual behavior; distortion of judgment and senses.	Statistical link to Kaposi's sarcoma (KS, an AIDS-related cancer); suspected immuno-suppression.
PSYCHEDELIC (LSD, mushrooms, etc.)	Usually caused by impurities, such as strychnine; few direct effects due to low quantity of chemical; early reports of chromosome damage unverified.	Severe alterations in perception and judgment; possible psychosis, mental instability; conducive to high risk-sexual activity; extreme suggestibility.	Unknown.
SPEED (crystal, amphetamines; most commonly injected)	Liver and heart damage; neuropathy (nerve damage); possible brain damage; weight loss; nutritional and vitamin depletion; adrenal depletion (uses up the body's energy reserves).	Distorted judgment, values, senses; delusions of strength; anxiety, paranoia, rebound depression; financial strain; powerful psychological addiction; conducive to high-risk sexual activity.	Likely immuno-suppression (not currently measured); potential for unknown and risky drug interactions; complication in treatment of brain disorders.
TOBACCO (cigarettes)	Several forms of lung disease, including lung cancer; cancers of the mouth; heart disease; arteriosclerosis; increased spread of skin cancers; extreme physical addiction.	Harm to others from second-hand smoke; bedroom burns; accidental fires; social rudeness; property damage.	Immuno-suppression; complications in treatment of lung diseases; increased frequency and severity of lung disease.

**STEP ONE:
WHERE AM I NOW?**

No one, certainly not this book, can demand that we give up all drug use to help combat AIDS. Yet, from a purely medical viewpoint, that is an easy case to make. For those with a dependency, total abstinence is the only possible solution. For others, any drug use or abuse constitutes some degree, however small, of added risk and strain on health or judgment. The choice of the individual is to determine just how much risk and strain is acceptable in return for the perceived benefits of drug use.

In the exercises which follow, you'll have an opportunity to accomplish several things:

- personally categorize your drug behavior, if any, as DEPENDENCY, ABUSE, or USE;

- informally assess the impact of drugs on the risk of spreading or contracting AIDS, and on the direct impact of each on your health;

- if you choose, set a goal and establish an action plan for changing drug behavior;

- explore the steps you might take to implement such a plan.

Dependency

Instructions:

Check off your responses to the questions below. These questions can help you decide if you or a person close to you may need help in dealing with drug dependency, including alcoholism. When you've finished, evaluate your scores using the Interpretation Guide at the end of the exercise.

		YES	NO
1.	Do you occasionally drink heavily or increase drug use after a disappointment, a quarrel or under stress at work?	☐	☐
2.	When you have trouble or are under pressure, do you always drink or use drugs more heavily than usual?	☐	☐
3.	Have you noticed that you are able to handle more drugs or alcohol than you did when you first began use?	☐	☐
4.	Did you ever wake up "the morning after" and discover you couldn't remember part of the evening before, even though your friends tell you that you did not "pass out"?	☐	☐
5.	When drinking or using drugs with others, do you have a few extra drinks or drugs others will not know about?	☐	☐
6.	Are there certain occasions when you feel uncomfortable if alcohol or drugs are NOT available?	☐	☐
7.	Do you sometimes feel a little guilty about your drinking or drug use?	☐	☐
8.	Are you secretly irritated when friends or loved ones discuss your drinking or drug use?	☐	☐
9.	Have you recently noticed an increase in the frequency of memory "blackouts"?	☐	☐
10.	Do you find you sometimes wish to continue drinking or using drugs after friends say that they've had enough?	☐	☐
11.	Do you usually have a "reason" for the occasions that you drink or use drugs heavily?	☐	☐

12. When you are sober or not using drugs, do you regret things you've done or said when drinking or using drugs? YES ☐ NO ☐

13. Have you tried changing types of liquor or drugs or tried different plans for controlling your consumption? YES ☐ NO ☐

14. Have you failed to keep promises you made to yourself or others about controlling or cutting down on your use of drugs or alcohol? YES ☐ NO ☐

15. Have you tried to control your drinking or drug use by making a change in jobs, friends, or relationships, or moving to a new location? YES ☐ NO ☐

16. Do you try to avoid family or close friends while drinking or using drugs? YES ☐ NO ☐

17. Are you having an increasing number of financial or work problems? YES ☐ NO ☐

18. Do more people seem to be treating you unfairly without good reason? YES ☐ NO ☐

19. Do you eat very little or irregularly when drinking or using drugs? YES ☐ NO ☐

20. Do you sometimes have "shakes" or get anxious in the morning and find that it helps to have a little drink or to use some drugs? YES ☐ NO ☐

21. Have you recently noticed that you can no longer drink or use as much drugs as you once did? YES ☐ NO ☐

22. Do you sometimes stay drunk or stoned for several days at a time? YES ☐ NO ☐

23. Do you sometimes feel very depressed and wonder whether life is worth living? YES ☐ NO ☐

24. Sometimes after periods of drinking or drug use do you see or hear things that aren't there? YES ☐ NO ☐

25. Do you get frightened easily after you have been drinking or using drugs heavily? YES ☐ NO ☐

(Based on a checklist by the National Council on Alcoholism)

The National Council on Alcoholism
12 West 21st Street
New York, NY 10010
(212) 206-6770

The National Council on Alcoholism
2655 Van Ness Avenue
San Francisco, CA
(415) 563-5400

INTERPRETATION GUIDE:

If you have answered "YES" to any of the questions, you have some of the symptoms that may indicate dependency or alcoholism. "YES" answers to several questions indicate the following stages of dependency or alcoholism:

Questions 1-8, early stages

Questions 9-21, middle stages

Questions 22-26, beginning of final stages

For additional information and related services, see the RESOURCES APPENDIX chapter of this book.

Medication and Prescription Drugs

Instructions:

Occasionally, people inadvertently begin to abuse medication prescribed by their doctor. This occurs when the prescribed strength and frequency does not seem adequate to the person to "control" worrisome symptoms, most commonly those of pain, anxiety and insomnia.

Check off each of the following conditions you may have noted while using tranquilizers, pain or sleep medication.

1. Feeling tired or having a clouded mental state.　　YES ☐　NO ☐

2. Feeling "hyperactive" or nervous.　　YES ☐　NO ☐

3. Anticipating my next dose ahead of time.　　YES ☐　NO ☐

4. Wishing for a higher dose or stronger medication.　　YES ☐　NO ☐

5. Supplementing medication with alcohol or drugs obtained from friends.　　YES ☐　NO ☐

6. Thinking of going to more than one doctor for medication.　　YES ☐　NO ☐

If you answered yes to any of these questions, it is possible that a problem is developing with your use of prescription medications. Your doctor may be able to suggest alternative ways of coping with anxiety, pain and insomnia while reducing or eliminating use and potential abuse of mind- or mood-altering medications.

The Dependency of Others

INSTRUCTIONS:

For each drug or alcohol dependent, at least four close friends or relatives *in addition* to the addicted person are adversely affected. Complete the following checklist to determine if you could benefit from help regarding the dependency of someone you care about.

1. Do you worry about how much someone else drinks or uses drugs? YES ☐ NO ☐

2. Do you have money problems because of someone else's drinking or drug use? YES ☐ NO ☐

3. Do you cover up someone else's drinking or drug use? YES ☐ NO ☐

4. Do you feel that if the drinker or drug user loved you, he or she would stop drinking to please you? YES ☐ NO ☐

5. Do you think that the drinker's or drug user's behavior is caused by his or her companions? YES ☐ NO ☐

6. Are routines frequently upset or meals delayed because of the drinker or drug user? YES ☐ NO ☐

7. Do you make threats, such as, "If you don't stop drinking or using drugs, I'll leave you"? YES ☐ NO ☐

8. When you kiss the addict hello, do you secretly try to smell his or her breath or look for signs of drug use? YES ☐ NO ☐

9. Are you afraid to upset someone for fear it will set off a drinking bout or increased use of drugs? YES ☐ NO ☐

10. Have you been hurt or embarrassed by a drinker or drug user's behavior? YES ☐ NO ☐

11. Does it seem as if holidays are spoiled because of drugs?   YES ☐   NO ☐

12. Have you considered calling the police for help for fear of violence or abuse?   YES ☐   NO ☐

13. Do you find yourself searching for hidden liquor or drugs?   YES ☐   NO ☐

14. Do you often ride in a car with a driver who has been under the influence of drugs?   YES ☐   NO ☐

15. Do you refuse social invitations out of fear or anxiety?   YES ☐   NO ☐

16. Do you sometimes feel like a failure when you think of the lengths you have gone to control the addict?   YES ☐   NO ☐

17. Do you think that if the drinker or drug user stopped this behavior, your other problems would be solved?   YES ☐   NO ☐

18. Do you ever threaten to hurt yourself to scare the drinker or drug user?   YES ☐   NO ☐

19. Do you feel angry, confused, or depressed most of the time?   YES ☐   NO ☐

20. Do you feel that no one understands your problems?   YES ☐   NO ☐

If you answered yes to some of these questions, you may also benefit from contacting Al-Anon or a similar service agency which assists the friends and families of drug dependents. (See the RESOURCES APPENDIX of this book).

(Based on a questionnaire provided to the public by the Al-Anon Family Group).

Quantifying Drug Effects

Instructions:

1. First, describe your health status with regards to the AIDS virus. Use this scale:

| Tested | Tested positive | Diagnosed | Diagnosed |
| negative | or unknown | ARC | AIDS |

   1 ------------------ 2 ------------------- 3 -------------------- 4

Tested negative =	taken the test and found to be negative.
Positive/unknown =	taken the test and found to be positive, or simply haven't taken it.
ARC =	diagnosed as having an AIDS-Related Condition.
AIDS =	diagnosed as having AIDS.

2. FOR EACH DRUG LISTED on the following page WHICH YOU USE:

   A. In COLUMN A, give the approximate date of the last time you used the drug.

   B. In COLUMN B, list how often you use the drug; use whichever of these scales fits best: times per month, or times per week, or times per day.

   C. In the box in column C, rate the overall impact of this drug use on your life on a scale from 1 to 5, including its financial, legal, and health effects. Use this scale to determine your rating:

   | Not harmful | | Somewhat harmful | | Very harmful |

   1 ------------- 2 --------------- 3 --------------- 4 -------------- 5

   D. In the box in column D, rate the degree to which you feel this drug use is "worth" whatever it is costing you. Take into account whatever pleasure you get from it, as well as whatever risks it is causing you. Use this scale to determine your rating:

   | Not worthwhile | | Somewhat worthwhile | | Totally worthwhile |

   1 ------------- 2 --------------- 3 --------------- 4 -------------- 5

	Last time used	**How often used**	**Impact (1-5)**	**Value (1-5)**
Alcohol	_____	_____	☐	☐
Cocaine	_____	_____	☐	☐
Downers	_____	_____	☐	☐
Hybrids	_____	_____	☐	☐
Marijuana	_____	_____	☐	☐
Opiates	_____	_____	☐	☐
Poppers	_____	_____	☐	☐
Psychedelics	_____	_____	☐	☐
Speed	_____	_____	☐	☐
Tobacco (cigarettes)	_____	_____	☐	☐

**STEP TWO:
WHERE DO I WANT
TO BE?**

Setting realistic goals for changing drug behavior requires knowing whether the problem is drug DEPENDENCY, ABUSE, or USE. When DEPENDENCY is involved, goal-setting can become a diversion, part of the path of denial. Many drug dependents go through a repeated cycle of promises of reform followed by failure to keep those promises. Every dependent has periods of sobriety in which the damage inflicted on self and others becomes evident. In such moments, addicts routinely and sincerely promise to make the needed changes, to quit, to stop causing the pain. The sincerity of the commitment makes it even more painful when the next binge begins. Loved ones are dragged along on a bruising roller coaster ride, wanting to believe in and support the next effort at reform, never wanting to give up hope. For the drug addict, goal-setting such as that described here only works in the context of getting help. Dependency, including alcoholism, is never kicked reliably through will power or even with the love of friends. Help is readily available through AA, physicians (who can recommend local resources), and gay-sensitive drug or alcohol treatment programs.

For ABUSE and USE, the goals also must begin with a clear understanding of the problem and a strong motivation to change. For many of us, AIDS has provided a new impetus to change. Drug behaviors we would have argued to protect only a short time ago now seem less defensible. In setting goals, we need to be clear that we're doing it for ourselves, for our own reasons—not as an admission that smug moralists were right all along. We need to look at change as something we do not for reasons of right or wrong, good or bad, but simply from the perspective of health. And, if it helps, we can do it with the understanding that we might have made different choices under different circumstances.

Although we can't help but face some degree of the "I told you so" syndrome from our critics, we have one sure satisfaction in changing our drug behaviors: we'll live a lot longer than they'd like.

Goal Setting

Instructions:

Using the space below, set your goals for changing drug behavior. List each drug and the behavior category your use falls into (USE, ABUSE, DEPENDENCY). If you're confronting DEPENDENCY in one area, don't ignore USE or ABUSE in another. Remember the characteristics of effective goals:

REALISTIC AND ACHIEVABLE
MEASURABLE AND OBSERVABLE
SET WITHIN TIME LIMITS

DRUG: _____
GOAL #1: _____
_____
_____

DRUG: _____
GOAL #2: _____
_____
_____

DRUG: _____
GOAL #3: _____
_____
_____

DRUG: _____
GOAL #4: _____
_____
_____

STEP THREE: HOW AM I GOING TO GET THERE?

The category of drug use largely determines the basic action plan needed. For example, DEPENDENCY requires help, period. To break out of DEPENDENCY requires not only the motivation and will to do so, but a replacement of the environment which supported the DEPENDENCY in the past. It is virtually impossible to give up a drug yet still be a part of the environment in which the addiction occurred. Alcoholics must find something to do with the time previously spent in bars or at home alone drinking. Crystal freaks, coke fiends, and junkies must find new types of people to associate with. Compulsive marijuana users must get out of the cloud of smoke. Cigarette smokers who quit often can't handle being in the presence of those who still smoke.

Groups such as Alcoholics Anonymous have long provided the social and psychological support needed to combat dependency. Most such groups even have gay chapters which offer an environment more comfortable for us and more sensitive to our needs. Help offered by a growing number of hospital clinics meets the need for some people and the cost is often covered by health insurance plans. For cigarette addicts, numerous options have opened up in the last several years as breaking the tobacco habit has become a business in itself.

Drug USE and ABUSE can also be most effectively overcome with professional help, especially if it is a long-standing problem. Some people, though, are able to bring drug USE and ABUSE under control with the help of friends, lovers, family, or support groups. Deciding which route to take calls for self-knowledge. A few questions to ask:

What has worked for you in the past?

How severe is the problem, how strong (or weak) is your motivation for overcoming it?

How critical is it to end the problem NOW? (Are there medical concerns? Is there damage to relationships or employment?)

How strong is your personal support system? Are you alone, without many close friends, or do you have many close friends, a lover who will help?

Another important consideration in establishing an action plan for making changes in drug behavior is how we plan to replace what we're giving up. It's safe to assume that drug use, appropriately or inappropriately, meets a need of some kind in our lives. Some needs commonly associated with drug use:

- relief from stress, to relax

- relief from sexual anxiety, guilt, internalized homophobia

- to loosen up, have fun, get crazy

- to overcome shyness, to socialize, be part of a group

- to get energized, to dance the night away

All of these are legitimate needs. If we've used drugs to meet them, we need to find another way if drug behavior is to be changed. All of them can be accomplished in other ways, ways which are less harmful to our health, less threatening in light of AIDS. For example:

NEED	ALTERNATE RESOURCE
Stress relief, relaxation	Massage; meditation; stress reduction techniques; more sex; vacation; nude bowling leagues.
Relieve sexual anxiety, guilt, internalized homophobia	Counseling; reading; support groups —confronting the problem rather than disguising it; dishing a friend who's *really* been bad.
Loosen up, have fun	Attitude, girl, it's all in your attitude; find a new crowd; try new things; shop; just get off it!
Overcome shyness, socialize	Social clubs; the gym; support groups; volunteer service; theater; public nudity; make a porno flick; join a jack-off club (you weren't planning to give up sex forever, were you?).
Energy	Exercise, fitness training; better diet; turn off the TV; pursue a new man.

Whatever we use drugs for in our lives, we can find a substitute if we want to. With few exceptions, drugs have only been a shortcut, one which really doesn't get us where we're going.

Action Plan

Instructions:

For each of the drug behavior goals established, describe an action plan for making change. Refer back to the page on which you established your goals, then work on this page to develop the ACTION PLAN. The plan should include three elements: (1) what kind of help, if any, you will seek in making change; (2) what steps you will take to get that help; and (3) a list of what you felt you were getting out of the drug use, and how you will meet that need in another way.

GOAL #1: Who will help? _____
_____

ACTION STEPS: _____
_____

What needs was the drug fulfilling?   How will you fulfill them without drugs?

_____   _____
_____   _____
_____   _____

GOAL #2: Who will help? _____
_____

ACTION STEPS: _____
_____

What needs was the drug fulfilling?   How will you fulfill them without drugs?

_____   _____
_____   _____
_____   _____

GOAL #3: Who will help? _____

_____

ACTION STEPS: _____

_____

What needs was the drug fulfilling?   How will you fulfill them without drugs?

_____   _____

_____   _____

_____   _____

GOAL #4: Who will help? _____

_____

_____

ACTION STEPS: _____

_____

What needs was the drug fulfilling?   How will you fulfill them without drugs?

_____   _____

_____   _____

_____   _____

154

Step 4: Implementation

Instructions:

In this last step, list 2 things: (1) any steps along the way you might use to measure your success in changing drug behavior, and (2) any rewards or consequences you might set for yourself as an incentive. Since drug use has a way of consuming expendable income, spending that money on yourself or in some other way makes for a very convenient reward system.

GOAL #1: Steps _____

_____

Rewards/consequences _____

_____

_____

GOAL #2: Steps _____

_____

Rewards/consequences _____

_____

_____

GOAL #3: Steps _____

_____

Rewards/consequences _____

_____

_____

The Social Impact of AIDS

Friendship Is Strong Medicine

Family Relations

Coming Out

Setting Limits

Facing AIDS in Friendship and in Love

CHAPTER

5

SOCIAL SUPPORT

INTRODUCTION

The support of friends, companions, and lovers has always been particularly important in gay culture. Most gay men, unlike their straight counterparts, are not the center of a traditional family grouping. We don't thrive on the affection and needs of our offspring, and fewer of us spend our lives in wedlock with a single mate. Our relations with our birth-families are sometimes strained. Yet we have the same powerful needs for human contact and support as anyone. To get it, we typically count on our friends. Even those of us who are happily committed to a lover retain strong bonds to our friends.

AIDS has placed great demands on our social support systems and has taken its toll on our energies, both as individuals and as a community. Many of us have been called on to extend our help, love and support to sick or grieving friends. A virtual army of dedicated volunteers and low-paid workers provides a vast array of services to our community. Public health workers, physicians, and politicians alike have noted the extent of our commitment and response. Seldom has a community risen to help its own with such selflessness and dedication.

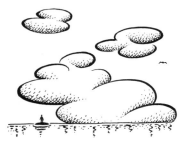

Social support—friendship, companionship, community, love, whatever we call it—is not important just for what it says about us. Coping with the fear or reality of AIDS is not the only reason why friends and support are important to our health. Friendship and warm personal contact have a significant *preventive* health role as well. Research has accumulated in recent years which paints a strong correlation between health and perceived support (the sense that there is "someone out there who is in my corner").

Two key aspects of social involvement are necessary to support our health: (1) an adequate number of contacts with other people (even if we don't have deep and profound interactions with all of them), and (2) the quality of our interactions and the degree of satisfaction we derive from them.

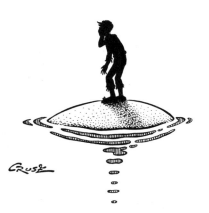

Human contact takes many forms. There is great variation in the ways people can love and relate to each other—our community has been a recognized leader in this regard. Relationships with lovers, with friends, and family can all provide opportunities for emotional dialogue, a sharing of feelings, desires, and needs. All are critical in helping us face the challenges that life presents, including the special challenges of AIDS.

The Social Impact of AIDS

Our concerns are substantial and undeniable these days, and thus our ability to count on each other—to be there for one another—must be up to the task. At least in regard to making and keeping friendships, a great many gay men report that the times have never been better. Many are finding this to be a time of greater openness with each other, a time to appreciate the more substantial and enduring aspects of our lovers, friends, families, and acquaintances. Yet, no one can deny that AIDS puts extra pressure on the social lives of everyone involved—people diagnosed, those who care for and about them, and those concerned about their own risks. A few common reactions, for better and for worse:

For better:

COMMUNION *(not the kind you get in church)*
Some people reach out to each other, sharing as never before their feelings, hopes, fears, and love. Long-time friendships blossom anew, the unspoken is spoken, and the things and people we truly cherish are acknowledged.

COMMITMENT *(the kind you see in AIDS organizations)*

Some devote time, money, and energy to helping others in need. Those who do often say they get more out of it than they can ever hope to give.

FAMILY RENEWAL *(soon to be a new sitcom)*
In times of crisis, it's natural to want to turn to our families. The birth-families we have often been so cut off from may now seek constant reassurance about our health *(yes, you, mother!)*. If we are ill, families (the caring kind) strive to renew or strengthen ties. Some, whose family ties were shattered by fear of disease and renewed homophobia, turn instead to the wonderful extended gay families which have evolved for many of us.

Or for worse:

WITHDRAWAL *(pulling out is always a downer)*
For some, involvement with others has become too difficult, too demanding, too risky; pulling back seems to be the only answer. Who among us was ever taught how to handle ourselves in a plague? Where did we learn how to support a friend who's just learned that he's dying? Isolation by choice, while easily understood, deprives us of the contact we need, and deprives others of the support they need from us.

SUPERFICIALITY *(who, me?)*
Some, after losing loved ones, find it too risky to care deeply again. Those who have lost many friends—and there are many—are especially prone to this. We avoid closeness and intimacy, afraid of being hurt again. Unfortunately, this doesn't make the pain go away. Instead, we are left feeling alone, even in a crowd.

FEAR AND HOSTILITY *(who asked you, buddy?)*
Under chronic pressure, some of us lose the ability to deal with others in a civil manner. The pain is so great for so long, that it is ready to break out at the slightest provocation. Some gay men have become afraid and angry at others or at the community, blaming it for the pain and suffering. Some fear that even safe contact is somehow risky.

SUPER-ACTIVITY *(gotta run; let's do lunch sometime)*
Some of us bury ourselves in a never-ending cycle of commitments and social events. Keeping constantly busy, whether in light-hearted social affairs or matters of deep commitment, may be a way of hiding from the horrors of the epidemic and its emotional impact. At the very least, it can prevent us from meeting our needs.

To face the challenges of AIDS, to meet our own needs and of those who count on us, we must find a balance, a path which permits us to get and give support.

FRIENDSHIP IS STRONG MEDICINE

Social relationships can have a profound and direct effect on our health. We've all heard the term "love sick"; many people believe that love also has the power to heal. Most of us have experienced the positive influence friends and family have on resolving our mental anxieties and depressions. Scientific research supports these views, at least in a general sense. The scientific case for the value of social contact is very strong:

- Both men and women have been found to be more susceptible to disease after the loss of a loved one.

- People in relationships experiencing conflict show temporary, measurable suppression of the immune system.

- Sociological studies show that as a part of involvement with others, we are more likely to engage in positive health behaviors such as exercise, medical check-ups, and health screening tests.

- In a study of older people, researchers found that having a *confidant* significantly helped people avoid psychiatric symptoms.

- Two studies of women showed that having an intimate and confiding relationship significantly reduced the incidence of depression.

- In a study of 7000 adults, a strong correlation was shown between social involvement and length of life; it was shown to be more important to health than smoking, drinking, exercise, or diet.

In these times, it is impossible to avoid some of the losses and separations that can affect our health negatively. It is also unreasonable to think that we can live a conflict-free existence. Yet, we can come to understand the impact that these powerful human events have upon us and make sure that we take extra measures to care for ourselves and others during these periods.

At the very least, social isolation—lack of the support provided by friendship—appears to be a predisposing condition for health deterioration. While science doesn't claim to prove that friendship can cure disease, most physicians will readily admit the patients with the best support often heal fastest.

FROM A MEDICAL PERSPECTIVE, social support helps to:

- maximize our resistance to disease;

- give us the best fighting chance if we are ill;

- assist others in attaining these same benefits.

FROM A SOCIAL PERSPECTIVE, other benefits emerge:

- Friends help us feel good about ourselves as gay people; they reassure us that we belong and that it's O.K. to be who we are.

- Friends provide emotional support—someone to talk to about our thoughts and feelings.

- Friends help us in material ways—help us solve problems, give us advice, even lend us money; in the AIDS crisis, this kind of support is invaluable.

STEP ONE: HOW'S YOUR SOCIAL LIFE?

Social support is critical in coping with the challenges of the present era. If we are getting what we need in this regard, our defenses against disease are maximized. Likewise, if we are giving others what they need from us, their strengths are also maximized. If our social contact is inadequate, either in quantity or quality, a price is being paid in our overall health—and we should do something about it.

In this chapter, the first step on the road to a healthier future requires that we identify our social contacts. The exercise on the following page will provide an opportunity for you to list the people in your life and arrange them in order of their closeness to you. In later exercises, you will be asked to evaluate the quality of the relationships as well. If either is lacking, or you simply feel there's room for improvement, goal setting and action planning follow.

In completing the exercise, remember that our judgment about who's "in" and who's "out" can change from day to day:

> *"That bitch actually said that about me!? He's off the 'intimate dinner party' list for good, and barely hanging onto the Xmas card list."*

To compensate for temporal whimsy, you may wish to think about how the list should look on the average, throughout the last year instead of how you might feel at the moment.

Who's Who?

Instructions, PART ONE:

1. Using the lined space, quickly list the names of the people you have any kind of repeated, caring social contact with, people you have warm feelings for, people you feel comfortable with—from lovers to acquaintances. Don't worry about ranking them—just list them as they come to mind. You may wish to check your address book to loosen your memory, but you needn't list everyone whose phone number you've ever had (this is a book, doll, not a library!).

_____ _____ _____

_____ _____ _____

_____ _____ _____

_____ _____ _____

_____ _____ _____

_____ _____ _____

_____ _____ _____

_____ _____ _____

_____ _____ _____

_____ _____ _____

_____ _____ _____

_____ _____ _____

_____ _____ _____

_____ _____ _____

_____ _____ _____

_____ _____ _____

Instructions, PART TWO:

2.   Write your own initials in the innermost circle of the rings on the next page (after all, we *are* the center of the universe, n'est pas?).

3.   Working from the list you created on the previous page, now place people in their actual positions on the diagram.

   List inside the ring closest to the center the initials of those with whom you feel the closest and most intimate bonds. People placed in this ring should all be of approximately equal closeness to you (though they may be close in different ways). For example, the closest circle might be reserved for your lover and/or for "best friends" if they are of about equal closeness. If you have an intense relationship with a lover who is closer to you in all ways than anyone else, who shares completely in your life, you might put him in the center circle along with yourself.

   Remember: this is about how *close* you feel to people, not how *often* you see them.

   Next, list the initials of those you feel the next closest to in the next outer ring, keeping people of approximately equal closeness in the same ring.

   Continue this process until you have placed all the people on your list in the appropriate circle.

NOTE: You may experience a sudden urge to get in touch with some of the people who come to mind. If so, don't interrupt the exercise to get on the phone (such an easy way to avoid completing the work). Instead, make a note to call them after you're finished.

Social Circles

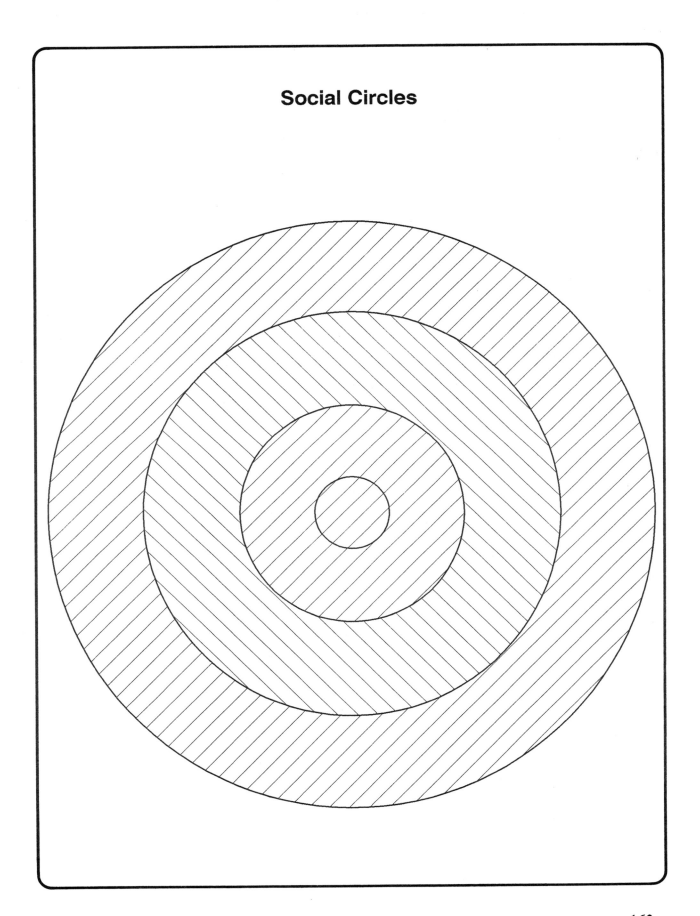

Instructions, PART THREE:

A. Add up your totals from the SOCIAL CIRCLES as follows:

     Number of people in circle 1 .... ☐

     Number of people in circle 2 .... ☐

     Number of people in circle 3 .... ☐

     Number of people in circle 4 .... ☐

B. Now make a separate count for the number of gay people, straight people you are fully out with, and straight people you are not out with.

     Gay people .... ☐

     Straight people I'm out with .... ☐

     Straight people I'm not out with .... ☐

(You may note how being out with people affects how close you feel to them. If some of the people you list in the innermost circles don't know you're gay, what does this say about those relationships? How close can you really be to someone who is unaware of this fundamental aspect of your identity?)

C. Now decide how you *feel* about what you see.

☐ Yes ☐ No   I have about as many friends as I can handle.

☐ Yes ☐ No   I'm satisfied with the distribution of my friends across the circles.

☐ Yes ☐ No   I'd like a different balance across the circles; specifically,

                   I'd like more friends in circle(s) ___ ___ ___

                   I'd like fewer friends in circle(s) ___ ___ ___

☐ Yes ☐ No   I'm just too popular! My public simply can't have all of me.

☐ Yes ☐ No   I've been hiding too long; I need more friends.

☐ Yes ☐ No   I have about as many gay friends as I would like (now, if they only *knew* they were gay!).

☐ Yes ☐ No   I have about as many straight friends as I would like.

☐ Yes ☐ No   I'm as close to and open with my family as I want to be.

In my own words, I feel: _____

_____

_____

_____

_____

_____

THE SUPPORT MAP

Looking at who our friends are and estimating their closeness to us tells only part of the story. Having a great number of friends can be wonderfully supportive, or it can be a tremendous drain on our strength and resources. Like ourselves, friends can both give and take. Each of us has a unique balance of giving and taking in our relationships, as do all of our friends. It may be in this balance between give and take, ours and our friends, that the net result on our health is determined.

We engage in friendship and social contact both to get our own needs met and to meet the needs of others. Although there is no single formula for achieving the proper give and take in a relationship, severe imbalances will almost always be harmful. Consider the possibilities:

ALL GIVE AND NO TAKE

This servantlike attitude, which has its roots in religious teachings and monastic practices, suggests that if we spend all our energy meeting the needs of others, somehow our own needs will automatically be met. This would be true if one's only need was to be needed by others. For the rest of us, all give and no take has little realistic appeal. We end up living our lives for others, and in doing so, lose any identity of our own. Over time, there is less and less, other than servitude, that we can truly contribute to others. Instead of finding that our needs will automatically be met, we quickly learn that others will let us be a doormat if that's what we seem to want. Like it or not, the nature of this world requires that we speak up for ourselves and ask for what we need. *People can't care about a guy who doesn't care about himself.*

ALL TAKE AND NO GIVE

At the opposite extreme is the "every man for himself" approach. It assumes that nobody ever does anything for anyone else—at least not without a good reason—and thus we'd better spend our energy looking out for good old number one. It's natural conclusion is insensitive and often cruel behavior which, in the end, interferes with our ability to get our needs met. While it's necessary and appropriate to look out for ourselves, our needs are best met with the willing cooperation of people who care about us. *People don't care about a guy who doesn't care about them.*

In between these extremes lie many levels of balance between giving and taking. Achieving a balance isn't easy under any circumstances and it is a real challenge in the shadow of AIDS. The levels of need and support that different people must present to each other in this crisis are sometimes seriously out of whack.

IF WE ARE ILL

Tremendous demands are made on our resources. Supplies of money, time, energy, patience—all typically diminish. There is less of each to go around, less to meet one's personal needs, through no fault of our own. Yet asking for help is very, very difficult. We may feel we are a burden or feel guilt and personal blame for being ill. Some of us look back in regret over every time in our lives when we didn't give fully to others. We are conditioned to feel that being in need somehow makes us weak, unmanly, or a failure. All of which is nonsense, of course. Still, many find that it is far more difficult to receive than to give.

The great traps: stubborn refusal to ask for, acknowledge, or accept the help we need; deliberate isolation; failure to recognize the many ways we can contribute in spite of (even because of) our disease.

IF WE ARE WELL

We experience less change in fundamental resources, yet may be called on to help in more ways than before, or to help more friends than before. Yet our resources are also limited. No one ever taught us how to help so many friends in need, how to lend a hand without patronizing. While our financial and energy resources may be stronger than those of our friends who are ill, we may face limits in our emotional and spiritual resources. We find ourselves frustrated, confused, and more than a little concerned about our own well-being.

The great traps: the Florence Nightingale syndrome (nurse to the masses); totally forgetting about our own needs (until we crack); well-meaning but insensitive attitudes (*"isn't it good of me to help you?"*); the Scrooge syndrome (*"let them help themselves"*).

Whatever gaps in resources develop in times of crisis, a realignment can always take place. Support can come in many forms; each of us has a way to give and a way to receive. To do either, we must do both.

Use the exercise on the following page to estimate the relative balance of give and take in your current relationships.

Give and Take

Instructions: (all apply to the chart on the following page)

1. In the column at the left, list the initials of the people you previously placed on your Social Circles diagram. Start with people in your innermost circles and work outward from there. You may wish to limit this to the people who are most important to you.

2. For each person, circle the letter which best describes the category of NEEDS which this relationship addresses. The need categories are as follows:

   A. Financial/practical matters

   B. Emotional support/love life (including loving sex)

   C. Entertainment/having fun (including recreational sex)

   D. Employment

   (For some people, you may circle all four categories if that is how you relate to each other).

3. In the next column, draw the symbol which best describes the RESULTS typically achieved in this relationship. When I have a problem, this person:

   + + Makes things a *lot* better   - - Makes things a *lot* worse

   + Makes things better   - Makes things worse

   = Even balance of better and worse

4. In the last column, describe the overall balance of GIVE AND TAKE in the relationship. Write a number in the box based on the scale below:

All give on my part		Balanced give and take		All take on my part
1 --------	2 ---------	3 ---------	4 --------	5

Person (initials)	Need Category	Results	Give and Take
_____	A B C D	[ ]	☐
_____	A B C D	[ ]	☐
_____	A B C D	[ ]	☐
_____	A B C D	[ ]	☐
_____	A B C D	[ ]	☐
_____	A B C D	[ ]	☐
_____	A B C D	[ ]	☐
_____	A B C D	[ ]	☐
_____	A B C D	[ ]	☐
_____	A B C D	[ ]	☐
_____	A B C D	[ ]	☐
_____	A B C D	[ ]	☐
_____	A B C D	[ ]	☐
	A B C D	[ ]	☐

5. Finally, reflect on the following questions:

What surprises did you find? _____

_____

What is your reaction to your ratio of give and take? _____

_____

How do you feel about your answers in the "results" column? _____

_____

_____

COMMUNITY PARTICIPATION

In a recent documentary entitled *Before Stonewall* gay men and lesbians discussed their lives in the 40's, 50's, and early 60's. We learned that an active, underground gay movement existed before most of us were born. We owe a great debt to these men and women who took those first precarious steps toward legitimizing our lives. In the past twenty years, our freedoms have expanded in many ways. We now have openly gay institutions and neighborhoods, we wield considerable political clout in some urban areas, and most of us feel far freer just to be ourselves. Yet, the social climate and freedom of expression still vary widely from one location to another and there is room for improvement even in the best of places. At worst, homosexuality is still a crime in many states and violence against gay people is on the rise even in our most liberated cities.

Some consider participation in the gay community to be an indicator of our comfort with our own gayness. It would be a mistake, however, to use it as an absolute measure, since many people who feel perfectly comfortable with their gayness travel in different circles and don't live a life that centers around being gay. Community involvement can be very helpful in coming to grips with our own sexuality as it provides a safe and supportive environment in which to explore our gay identities. In a world which routinely transmits homophobic messages, having a place where gayness is valued plays an important role in our self-development and self-acceptance. Community involvement—membership in gay organizations, joining or supporting gay causes, living near other gay people, shopping, socializing or dining in gay neighborhoods—provides opportunities to meet other gay people. In rap and support groups or consciousness raising activities, we can directly address and perhaps heal some of the wounds acquired while in the closet.

The gay community is perhaps the best place in the world to find support and up-to-date information for combating AIDS. Gay periodicals are an excellent source of medical information, and, as a bonus, they typically include political and social analysis (not to mention some very interesting ads and pictures). Gay resources on AIDS are so strong that teeming hordes of card-carrying heterosexuals now descend upon our hotlines and information services (there goes the neighborhood!).

Political action, another form of community involvement, plays a special role in gay life. As an oppressed group, acute political awareness and action are necessary for the mere survival of our community. Taking an active role in gay politics can give a sense of purpose and help reduce the sense of powerlessness we sometimes feel.

Lavender is a Color in the Rainbow

Membership in our community comes in all shapes, colors, and class backgrounds. Many of us have experienced multiple levels of oppression and discrimination. For example, our Black, Hispanic, and Asian brothers sometimes seem to get it from all sides. Unfortunately, our community hasn't always been as concerned as one would expect from a minority community. Charges of discrimination in hiring and admission have long been voiced against gay bars and clubs which try to promote a "certain image." As one man put it:

> *"We feel caught and rejected on both sides. Our families and the black church condemn us, and the gay community gives us a cold shoulder."*

Gay men with physical disabilities note a tendency toward what has been called "lookist" attitudes (similar to racist or sexist attitudes), a form of discrimination based on physical appearance or capability.

People, even gay people, seem to try awfully hard to find ways to decide who's *in* and who's *not*. This is a crude and hurtful practice, one that groups which are themselves subject to discrimination should certainly be above. As an emerging community in the process of defining itself, we have an opportunity to demonstrate new standards of acceptance and openness toward one another. As a group, we have a great deal to offer (and gain) in a growing alliance of people disenfranchised by the traditional majority. We owe it to all our brothers under the lavender rainbow to extend a friendly hand of welcome and support, a welcome which is blind to color, race, sex, ability, and economic or social class.

Living in the Ghetto

Yes, Barbra, sometimes enough is truly enough. In some cities we can literally insulate ourselves within the gay community. We can live in a gay neighborhood, work for a gay establishment, shop only in gay stores, go to a gay doctor, and expect to see a gay man when we call the police. In the Castro District in San Francisco, it is said that only gay people are sent out to repair the phones. Similar situations exist in major cities throughout the country—the Village and Christopher Street in New York, West Hollywood, the Sheffield district in Chicago, and the Montrose area in Houston are just a few examples.

While living in a gay fantasyland may seem like nirvana, a variety of problems are sometimes associated with these gay paradises. Certainly, the devastation of AIDS has been hastened in the most insular neighborhoods—it almost couldn't be otherwise. Isolation may also reinforce the view that the outside world is a dangerous place (which at times it may be). To outsiders, gay neighborhoods seem to be forbidden lands populated by strange beings—heterosexual imaginations run wild, envisioning men in dresses and leather daisy-chained around fire hydrants.

There are clearly some benefits in mixing things up with the non-gay population—for us and for them. Adaptability is a key element in any group's survival; a group as threatened as ours might benefit from this skill. As gay people, we must not settle for feeling welcome only in our own enclaves. We have a right to everything that society offers.

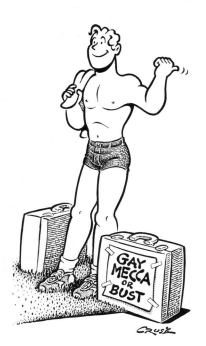

The great coastal gay meccas play host to thousands of gay men and women who have fled homes elsewhere in the country. An initial period of indulgence in the gay community is common. As one hunk put it, *"It was like I died and went to Gay Heaven."* Even AIDS hasn't changed this: in the old days, it was *"so many men, so little time";* today, it's *"so many groups, so many meetings."* After the initial excitement wears off, people often venture out into the rest of world, where heterosexuals are known to roam freely in the streets. We have a right to our freedom in the rest of the city as well.

Knowing there is a place to return to where we can fully be ourselves, a place to refuel and prepare to face another day—a safe haven—is more important than ever in these times. This security may be found in our homes or in a supportive gay community. With it, we find the courage to go into the world and be who we are.

To finish your assessment of *"where you are now,"* complete the following exercise, which assesses your level of community involvement.

Community Participation

Instructions:

A. In the boxes provided, check each of the following that you do and estimate how often (on the line).

		Gay	Non-gay
1.	Participate in community organizations	☐ _____	☐ _____
2.	Go to social clubs	☐ _____	☐ _____
3.	Participate in athletic events	☐ _____	☐ _____
4.	Participate in musical or artistic groups	☐ _____	☐ _____
5.	Have friends visit in your home or go to theirs	☐ _____	☐ _____
6.	Go to resorts	☐ _____	☐ _____
7.	Go to classes in which openly gay men are involved	☐ _____	
8.	Read gay papers or magazines	☐ _____	

B. Describe how you feel about your level of involvement with the gay community (check all that apply).

☐ Gay for days; hardly a non-gay minute in the week

☐ An even balance of gay involvement and other types

☐ Not involved in the gay community—by my own choice

☐ Not involved, or minimally involved; throbbing for change

☐ Don't see things in a gay/non-gay way

☐ No opportunity for involvement locally (but working to bring the local cowboys out)

FAMILY RELATIONS

AIDS has changed the family relations of many gay men for better and for worse. For some of us, who were able to come out to our parents before AIDS, a dialogue had already begun and AIDS was just another topic. Others have faced the agonizing double burden of telling their parents they were gay at the same time they were telling them they had AIDS.

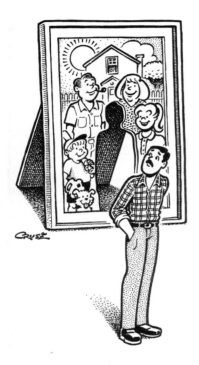

Understanding AIDS and its impact on our lives is challenging enough for ourselves; it is an enormous struggle for our families, especially if they haven't already accepted our gayness. We need to think carefully about what we want to tell them, how to go about it, and how they are likely to react. While blunt honesty might seem easiest, AIDS is so complex and frightening for them that a harsh dose of reality may be too much to take all at once. In addition to anxiety about our health, other hidden concerns can come to the surface—fear of infection, anger at the gay community, *"I told you so...,"* God's punishment and so on. Just about anything the general public has felt or heard about AIDS is a likely subject of conversation. At the extreme, the issue of AIDS has driven families apart, resulting in emotionally charged confrontations between the family and our lovers and friends. Families who long ago broke ties over a son's gayness have sometimes reappeared and reasserted their dominance and control, driving lovers from the bedside (and the homes and property acquired together). For some, it has been the last straw in an already crumbling relationship.

Yet, most family relationships have fared well in the face of AIDS. Many gay men, some sick, some well, report that warm and moving experiences have resulted. AIDS has brought many gay men together with their birth-families and repaired bonds that were broken long ago. For some, tolerance has grown into loving acceptance and understanding. Whatever the reaction, gay men and their families have responsibilities to each other in times of crisis such as this. Our families are unlikely to have a better source of accurate, unbiased information about AIDS than we ourselves can offer them. When we are ill or facing the uncertainties of AIDS, someone has to help the family understand and respect the importance of our lovers and friends—if necessary, to set things straight and put the family in its desired legal and emotional place. We alone, as their children, have the power to do so. Whatever direction things flow, it's up to us to lead the way. Those who have AIDS or any level of HIV infection need to let their families in on it, at least if there is any kind of a relationship going on. Those of us who aren't ill may need to talk with our families just to allay their unspoken fears in the crisis.

Can We Talk?

Instructions:

Check off the phrase which best describes your family situation.

OUR DISCUSSION OF AIDS:

☐ We haven't discussed it all.

☐ We've discussed it in general, not personal, terms.

☐ We've discussed my personal health status.

☐ We've discussed how AIDS has affected my life, the losses I've experienced, my feelings about it.

WHAT I MIGHT WANT TO TELL THEM:

☐ I want them left alone and the topic avoided (*"You don't know my mother!"*).

☐ I want them to have accurate information about the disease and who is at risk but not to be overly inquisitive about my own situation.

☐ I want them to know what my health status is at present and what risks I face.

☐ I'd like to discuss what is happening to me and my community—and I hope they're interested.

HOW I WANT THEM TO RESPOND:

☐ I want things to return to the status quo (*"Hi Dad, Hi Mom. Love the new curtains. See you next week."*).

☐ I want them to become better informed about the disease and the epidemic (*"No, you needn't wash the toilet seat after I go home"*).

☐ I want them to express genuine concern for my health (but without lecturing me on my lifestyle).

☐ I want increased emotional support from them.

☐ I want material or financial assistance from them (with no strings attached).

**STEP TWO:
WHERE DO I WANT
TO BE?**

In matters of social support, more is not always better. Increasing social involvement with friends and family can add demands as well as resources. Each of us must look at the degree of social support currently at hand, the balance of give and take, and decide for ourselves if we need to increase or decrease contact, or change the balance or quality of our relationships.

Some possible situations which might call for a goal for change:

-   if we feel isolated, alone, or lacking in friends or family ties

-   if our social calendar is loaded, but our relationships lack depth

-   if we fear that we don't have adequate social resources for meeting the demands we face (or might face if we become ill)

-   if our relationships with family members are less than open, less than supportive, less than honest

-   if we're wrapped up in activities, however worthwhile, in a constant state of giving and doing for others, yet somehow dying inside

-   if our friends are in need and we haven't been there to help

-   if we're wrapped up in ourselves—and no one really cares

-   if we're drifting away, a bit at a time, from all the people who used to matter

-   if we're dissatisfied living a lie—at work or among friends—about who we are, or if illness is forcing us out of the closet

-   if we can't achieve other goals for personal growth because they aren't supported by the crowd we run with

-   if AIDS has taken a lover or friend, or devastated our social circle

-   if we cry alone at night for no special reason

For any of these reasons, a goal for change might be appropriate. Goals may address at least the following:

-   an increase or decrease in the number of friends, in total or in one of the particular social circles

-   a change in the depth, quality, or subject matter of a relationship

-   a change in position with our natural family, friends, or co-workers, such as coming out or being more honest about a health situation

-   a change in the give and take in any or all of our relationships

-   an end to an unproductive, draining relationship

-   a change in our level of involvement in the gay community

Goal Setting

Instructions:

Using the space below, set up to four goals for making changes in your social situation. List each situation you wish to address, what you want to change about it, and when you're going to do it. Remember the characteristics of effective goals:

REALISTIC AND ACHIEVABLE
MEASURABLE AND OBSERVABLE
SET WITHIN TIME LIMITS

Situation: _____
GOAL #1: _____
_____
_____

Situation: _____
GOAL #2: _____
_____
_____

Situation: _____
GOAL #3: _____
_____
_____

Situation: _____
GOAL #4: _____
_____
_____

STEP THREE: HOW AM I GOING TO GET THERE?

Goals for change in our social support systems are particularly challenging since they involve the response of others as well as ourselves. No instant formulas can suddenly produce more friends, better or more relationships with family members, co-workers, or casual acquaintances. All of these changes take time. Before establishing an action plan for reaching your goals, consider the following extended discussion of the issues of friendship and how we can cope best with them. Much of the information which follows may be helpful in deciding just how to to make and implement changes in the social support system.

More on the Give and Take

Whether the context is love, affection, or material assistance, relationships which have an inherent balance between giving and taking seem to work more smoothly than those which don't. Exactly how the balance is achieved, however, is not always easy to recognize. Balance doesn't necessarily mean that each partner puts in an equal amount of the same things or at the same time. In many relationships, one partner has greater strengths in one area while the other is stronger in another. Differing strengths can complement each other and produce a workable balance.

Proper balance in a relationship does not occur spontaneously or by magic. We must be able to communicate about what is needed on an ongoing basis since our needs change so frequently:

- Often, we must let a friend or lover know what our needs are and when they aren't being met (*"Who me, need attention? Whatever gave you that idea? I often burst into tears for no apparent reason, don't you?"*)

- At times, we must ask a friend or lover to back off, to withhold some of their attention lest we be smothered by the relationship (*"Do you think maybe I could go into the bathroom alone, just this once, hon?"*)

- Sometimes, we must ask a friend or lover to ask a little less of us when we just don't have enough to give (*"Sorry, I just can't handle another crisis today. Can it possibly wait 'til morning?"*)

Learning to negotiate in relationships so that we both get what we want is an important skill, one which doesn't come automatically for anyone. It has three basic components:

1. BEING CLEAR ABOUT OUR OWN NEEDS and effectively communicating them.

2.   STRIVING TO UNDERSTAND THE NEEDS OF A FRIEND or partner (easy only if he or she is also good at step one above).

3.   SEEKING A BALANCE which takes both sets of needs and priorities into consideration.

In short, we need to understand both sets of needs—ours and our friend's—before we can find a successful balance. It isn't enough to assume that each partner will look out for his or her own side of the relationship. The old adage "looking out for number one" can be a good thing if it reminds us to communicate our own needs, but when it becomes the only rule, it will always upset the balance. We can't always count on each partner to be equally assertive about needs. Negotiating effectively requires that we look out for the needs of our partner as well as our own.

Setting Limits

One definition of love is the ability to place another's well-being before our own. In a prolonged crisis such as AIDS, many of us are asked to do this on a regular basis. Yet, for our own mental and physical health, we must periodically reevaluate our degree of involvement and commitment. If the demands are strong and frequent, we can easily burn out or give so much that our own needs go unmet. This may sound cold-hearted, but if it saves a relationship, the final effect is positive. We must ask ourselves, *"What am I willing to do? How much time can I devote to my friend who is in need?"* By being clear with loved ones, they will be able to set reasonable expectations and divide their support appropriately. The person in need will usually appreciate this since almost no one likes to ask too much.

Coming Out to the Family

However risky it might appear, coming out to the family can be a positive experience. Until the final moment when it happens, we each have a million reasons why we shouldn't—*"it will only cause them grief in their old age"; "my (mother) (father) will never understand"; "what's the point?"* and so on. Yet hundreds of thousands, perhaps millions of men and women have done it before, and only a few claim to regret it. If we choose to take the plunge, a few guidelines are in order to make it easier on both parties:

• PICK A COMFORTABLE TIME AND PLACE. Allow enough uninterrupted time to answer questions and discuss the matter, but set a limit so the discussion won't be endless. After a point, parents need time alone to let it sink in.

- KNOW IN ADVANCE WHAT YOU WANT TO SAY (*and what you don't*) in the first discussion. First rule: KISS (*Keep It Simple, Stupid*). Avoid discussing sexual practices or the finer points of gay life. Stick to the basics: how long you've known, why or how it has been good for you, whether or not you have a partner (*but don't bring him along*), why you haven't told them until now. Give them a positive, hopeful picture of gay life—the way it really is. If you don't have such a picture, see a counselor. If there's something they must know about your health status, prepare a description in advance (*rather than just blurting it all out*); remember, their understanding of AIDS issues may well be primitive.

- PROVIDE SUPPORTIVE READING (*even if your parents aren't the reading type*). There are several good books on the subject, books to help parents accept their gay children, books which describe famous, positive gay figures throughout history, books which deal with religious concerns about homosexuality (a few titles are listed in the *Resources Appendix* of this book). Most parents are delighted to learn that religious views on homosexuality are far from one-sided and have changed constantly throughout history. Buy them a pair of books you think they'll find helpful (*don't invite them to go browsing in a gay bookstore right away—they may not understand everything they find*).

- PLAN FOR THEIR SUPPORT. Before talking, pick out a brother, sister, another family member, or a friend who is close to them. Tell the other person what you are going to do (*but don't ask permission*), and ask him/her to be around to support them afterwards. Parents usually need to talk to someone about it, but often feel too embarrassed (*"Good grief, mother!"*) to bring it up with anyone. If you know friends of theirs who are sympathetic to gay people, or who have a gay son or daughter of their own, enlist their help.

- SET LIMITS FOR THE CONVERSATION. Refuse to allow the conversation to deteriorate into a shouting match. If it crosses that line, be prepared to politely end the discussion and come back another time. But leave the books anyway.

- DON'T ALLOW THEM TO BLAME THEMSELVES. Parents love to play the old *"where did we go wrong"* game. The answer: NOBODY went wrong, not them, not you. Gayness is a naturally occurring variation of human sexuality, it is common throughout nature. It is not a matter of choice, nor is it because of anything they did or did not do. It just IS, like the color of the sky, like their own sexuality (*or anyone else's*). Everything you are, everything that's good about you, remains. Nothing is changed except their knowledge of who catches your eye when you walk down the street, who you'd like to share your bed or your life with.

- BE PREPARED TO DESCRIBE WHY YOU'RE TELLING THEM. No, it's not to make them suffer, or to be ashamed before their friends. Why then? Because you want them to know so they can love you as you really are. And you want them to have a positive attitude toward gay people in general (*because, as the saying goes, "we ARE your children"*).

- EXPECT TO BE SURPRISED. Vast numbers of gay men, after agonizing over this issue, find that their parents knew or suspected all along and have long since accepted the fact.

Going Public

In the same way that AIDS often pushed many of us out of the closet with our families, it has forced many into a similar disclosure in places of employment and among old friends, schoolmates, relatives, and neighbors. Those who are ill, who are caring for ill friends, or who have lost friends and lovers can't always keep it hidden. Discussion of AIDS, almost always linked to discussion of gayness, is virtually an epidemic in itself. Time and again we are asked to decide how far out of the closet we want to go, how far out is healthy for us to go.

Of course, the only "politically correct" answer is *all the way out.* Yet the price for doing so is as high, or higher, than ever before. Employers, insurance companies, ill-informed relatives, among others, have been known to take hard positions against gays these days. Yet the powerful impact of more and more people coming out is undeniable. In a way, gay people won't be truly free until none of us has anything to hide. Realistically, however, we aren't all crusaders. It's not unreasonable to look at the personal risks, weigh them against the benefits, and make our own decision. Participation in the gay community doesn't require that we all make the same choices. We do a disservice to each other to demand that everyone fall in line with our own views.

Whether the coming out occurs at places of employment, in the neighborhood, or among relatives, a constant theme of benefits apply.

- By learning that we are gay, people who already know and respect us will be forced to reconsider any possible biases or homophobia they harbor toward gay people as a group (a few, no doubt, will find it easier to reconsider their respect for us).

- We almost always experience a sense of relief from the ability to be fully ourselves in a wider circle.

- We often discover that people whose rejection we feared come to respect us more for our honesty and integrity.

- Many people who knew all along feel closer to us once we give them permission to acknowledge our gayness (*just who did you think you were fooling anyway, Bernice?*).

- Even critics sometimes respect our courage and reconsider their own stereotypes of gay people as a group (*"Him, a queer? You could'a fooled me"*) (and we've been doing it for years, Einstein).

- Elaborate ruses and deceptions are no longer necessary (no need to leave the *Playboy* on the coffee table, no fear of dressing *too* sharply, no need to mess up the apartment before the guys from work stop over).

- Coming out, under any circumstance, almost always feels better than we thought and brings with it a few pleasant surprises (like a date with that handsome guy who was trying so hard to convince you that he was straight).

The process of coming out to people in general is simpler than the model described for parents and family. We don't owe anyone an explanation of who we are or why. In fact, it's the other way around: they owe us unquestioned, unbiased acceptance (not mere tolerance). We have the same fundamental rights shared by all others, without regard to race, color, sex, beliefs, or sexual preference. We must demand it for ourselves, and give it freely to all others.

Coming Out to Ourselves

Coming out to ourselves is perhaps most difficult for our youngest brothers, who, just as they first accept their own growing sexual desires, quickly find those desires linked to illness and death. It used to be that any young gay man had little trouble finding men to teach him the ways of our world. Today, there is less opportunity for experimentation and fewer people willing to help. Learning to freely express our gay desires was always difficult—today it is even more so.

As a community we owe it to our younger (or later blooming) brothers to assist by providing ways for them to experiment in a safe and self-affirming manner. New institutions in our community—clubs, service groups, political organizations—make the unsafe alleyways and restrooms of our past turn into fond memories. As we recognize young or reluctant brothers straddling the line, our first thoughts must be of compassion rather than pity or exploitation. Crossing over is more difficult in this time than it was just a few years back. In short, we must help them see that being gay is natural and that they can live happy and fulfilled lives in spite of AIDS. They aren't getting this message from the rest of the world. Most importantly, we are obliged to teach them how to survive. Every hawk must teach his chickens to use rubbers; each daddy must instruct his students in the ways of safety; and each who has the opportunity must patiently teach our wedded brothers from the suburbs what's OK and what's not.

Relationship Styles

In the decade of the sexual revolution, some gay men prided themselves on the quantity of their relationships. While numbers certainly kept them busy, many reported little satisfaction in constant "scoring," long before AIDS began to exact its toll. These days, we are working hard to develop the quality of our relationships. To the casual observer, that may seem to be only a response to AIDS; an in-depth examination, however, shows that we are just as concerned with getting more out of our relationships, even relationships which are primarily sexual.

There are no widely accepted universal formulas for building relationships. Each of us must develop our own relationship style which takes into account our likes and dislikes, strengths and weaknesses, our quirks and endearments. To a great extent, it is our uniqueness which others find attractive.

Building a relationship style begins by examining our attitude toward ourselves. As gay people living in a homophobic society, coming to feel good about ourselves requires letting go of past hurts and grudges, forgiving ourselves for our own weaknesses and failures, and learning to recognize what's good, what's likable about ourselves. Until we do this, it will be difficult to develop satisfying relationships with others. Problems of fundamental self-acceptance cannot be solved by friendship alone. Many people find help in counseling and support groups. Friendship plays an important role, though, by providing a better understanding of the good others see in us.

Similarly, loving others requires that we give them the space they need to see their own self-worth. We carry an unfair burden of self-doubt and hatred from the homophobia drummed into us since childhood. While we must struggle with it personally, we can also make an effort to give each other a special break, always extending just a little more understanding and forgiveness than the world has given us.

This takes courage and determination, especially if past experiences with others haven't gone well.

When we consistently find that others decline our interest in friendship, or don't seem to want to talk with us, it may be a sign that something we're doing turns people off. Blaming our looks, social standing, or other external factors is a cop-out, since there are people of all shapes, sizes, appearances, and status who have strong friendships. Often, it's something as simple as how we conduct a conversation. A few tips on the art of conversation which ease the path to friendship:

LISTEN ACTIVELY (give others your undivided attention)
So many of our conversations sound like contests. While one guy talks, the other is preparing his next remark. Yet neither is really listening to the other. Is there a gay man anywhere who hasn't taken part in conversations like these? What they convey is a lack of interest and concern for the other person. Yet, we do it all the time, even with valued friends. The easiest way to break the habit is to make a point of asking simple questions of the guy who is speaking, questions which delve a little deeper into what he is saying. This communicates real interest and concern, and makes it easier for him to open up. *Doesn't it feel good when someone truly listens to you?*

ASSUME VALUE (look for the positive)
Perhaps because of the negativity we have experienced ourselves, many of us have a tendency to instinctively look for what's wrong with other people. Gay people have made a fine art of dishing one another, and while it's mostly in jest, a lot of unseen pain is often the result. Friendship grows more easily in a climate of support and agreement, rather than criticism and cutting retorts. Make an effort to first look for what's good in other people; look, listen, and speak from as positive a perspective as you can. Most of our judgments are arbitrary anyway, so why lead with our claws? *In short, give a girl a break—there's always plenty of time to read her beads later.*

EXPRESS AGREEMENT & GOOD FEELINGS (don't just think it)
Although we often feel positive things about friends and new acquaintances, we tend to be overly shy or forgetful about expressing them. If you like the way someone looks, talks, thinks, or dresses, say so. Even among long-time friends, we seldom say how much we mean to each other. This works in both ways—as we become more expressive with others in a positive way, they instinctively do so with us. Wouldn't it be nice to take the artificially harsh edge

off so many of our gay conversations? *Do we have to carry on like like Rex Reed burying a bad movie?*

These simple steps are not big news, since we instinctively use them when courting our latest dream man. The key to making them work for improving our relationships in general is simply to become aware of them and use them deliberately and regularly. With a little practice, they become a habit.

Intimacy

Intimacy is the experience of allowing another person to know us on a deep level. This may be the result of long association or it may be sudden and spontaneous. In moments of intimacy we seem to blend together with the other person. We are as one. For some, orgasm is the only route to this profound sense of togetherness (while for others, orgasm can only occur in the absence of personal intimacy). Others are able to find different avenues to this profound experience, for example, deep and emotional conversation or mutual involvement in strongly valued activities such as music or political activity.

Intimacy must grow out of mutual consent—it cannot be forced no matter how badly we desire it. One-sided attempts at intimacy put great strains on a relationship and drive people apart. Either you both get there together, or you don't get there at all. People vary in their capacities for intimacy and their interest in it at any particular time. Some, after experiencing such a moment, feel uncomfortable and draw away from the other person. Some psychologists believe that our capacity for intimacy is closely associated with our sense of self-worth and acceptance. If we don't feel good about ourselves down deep, intimacy can be frightening. It leaves us feeling that others will discover our inadequacy, our worthlessness. Successful experiences of intimacy, on the contrary, reassure us that we are good and worthy of love despite our imperfections. Developing our capacity for intimacy is a life-long pursuit, one which is closely related to the quality of our relationships.

Finding a Lover

With the renewed interests in long-term relationships we are experiencing as a community, we might expect that this would be an excellent time for finding a lover. While the interest may be there, so too is increased fear of intimacy and loss. On the bottom line, this era is perhaps no better or worse than any other for finding a lover.

Seeking a lover as a way to find safe and reliable sex may well be a futile pursuit. The sex may be neither safe nor reliable, though the expectations will certainly be high. Good relationships can only be built upon solid foundations, not on fear and anxiety. A relationship begun today should have the same cornerstones of mutual interest, affection, intimacy, and compatibility as at any other time. Relationships begun today, however, do have some special requirements. Both parties, for example, must be honest and up front about their health status. A sense of each other's sexual history is important as a reference point for sexual safety within the relationship. Each person's interest in or commitment to monogamy must be known if unprotected sex is envisioned (after adequate and repeated testing). We owe each other complete honesty in these matters. A relationship which begins without it is certain to fail.

Since long nights at the bar are less common these days, other opportunities for meeting people must be utilized. Many people feel the best time and place to meet a lover is when our attention is focused outside of ourselves. Community organizations provide excellent meeting grounds, as do places of work and recreation. When we meet someone of interest, the early stages of the relationship are best directed at finding common interests, shared activities, and joint pursuits. Moving too quickly on the emotional front, seeking early commitments, and expecting too much too soon are guaranteed ways to throw water on the fire. It's often easy to recognize when the time comes to make commitments—you'll notice that you've both been living as if they were already made.

A secure and lasting relationship is a treasure for anyone, gay or straight. It must be pursued with respect—not desperation—and nurtured with love and selflessness. The specter of AIDS changes neither our need for such relationships nor our capacity to engage in them.

Action Planning

Instructions:

Refer back to the social support goals you wrote out several pages back in this chapter. Briefly restate each goal below and then develop an ACTION PLAN for achieving it. Incorporate the suggestions made in this chapter on coming out and improving the quality of relationships.

The plan should include two elements: (1) what STEPS you will take to make the changes identified by your goals; (2) what RESOURCES you will call on for help, if needed.

GOAL #1: _____

_____

ACTION STEPS: (what are you going to do, and when) _____

_____

_____

_____

_____

RESOURCES or strategies you will apply: _____

_____

_____

_____

GOAL #2: _____

_____

ACTION STEPS: _____

_____

_____

_____

RESOURCES or strategies you will apply: _____

_____

_____

GOAL #3: _____

_____

ACTION STEPS: _____

_____

_____

_____

RESOURCES or strategies you will apply: _____

_____

_____

GOAL #4: _____

_____

ACTION STEPS: _____

_____

_____

_____

RESOURCES or strategies you will apply: _____

_____

_____

FACING AIDS IN FRIENDSHIP AND IN LOVE

Few experiences in life match the intensity of a face-to-face encounter with death. When watching someone we love suffer from AIDS, we experience mankind's most profound emotions. For our community, this has become an all too frequent experience. As one man bereaving the loss of his lover poignantly stated, *"At least he gets to die, I'm left behind to live with his loss."*

Sharing the experience of facing a life-threatening illness with another person can be both a privilege and a profound growth experience. Much is asked of us, much is taken from us, and much is given to us. At times it can drive the strongest of us to our limits. As gay men, we may be called upon to face AIDS on several possible levels, for our friends or lovers, or ourselves:

- coping with a positive response on the AIDS antibody test

- coping with a diagnosis of ARC or the early stages of AIDS

- coping with a diagnosis of full-blown AIDS

- coping with the final days and loss of a loved one

Each situation places its own burden on the relationship. After the initial shock of any of these situations, our relationships must settle into a changed pattern which adjusts to the new reality. New demands may be made; a delicate balance may be upset and will certainly be changed. New pressures may exist as emotions are strained. Both parties in the relationship, the one who receives the diagnosis and the one who stands by his side, face unique new challenges. Great sensitivity and care will be asked of each. Sometimes, as we know, both partners may be struck at once.

Though there are no simple solutions to ease these tremendous burdens, some steps can be taken to make the best of a bad situation. From the suggestions which follow, use whichever seem most appropriate and helpful. Recognize, however, that the issues are so profound, so extensive, that most people seek professional or group support to help in coping.

Coping with AIDS Antibody Testing

Coming to terms with antibody testing is for many the first step in a long process of making medical decisions related to AIDS. From the beginning, friends can be of immeasurable help in deciding what to do and giving support. Antibody testing should not be considered without clear information about what the test's result means, what are its limitations, and the potential risks and benefits it provides to the person being tested (this issue is discussed further in the *Fighting For Our Lives* chapter of this book). Friends can be very helpful in gathering this information and helping us think it through. The opinions of friends are not, however, a substitute for informed and sensitive medical assistance.

Additional support is, of course, needed if we receive a positive test result. Calm review with a friend can be a big help in deciding what, if anything, to do about the test outcome. Reassurance of continued support will help reduce the fear of the unknown that accompanies such tests. With each passing year, we learn more about what a positive antibody test means—discussing the situation with friends can help us keep abreast of the latest interpretation. If we take a particularly hopeless view of the implications, knowledgeable friends can help us see also that much progress is being made toward treatment, especially for people in early stages of the illness.

Helping friends cope with the test and its implications is an important responsibility, one which shouldn't be taken lightly. If we offer our advice and opinions, we'd better know what we're talking about. Yet, we can be of great assistance without being an expert on the test itself. Helping a friend admit to his fear, sadness, or rage may be more valuable than anything else we can offer. To help a friend at a moment like this, a few tips might be helpful:

BEFORE THE TEST:

- SHARE YOUR VIEWS, but don't debate his. To test or not to test is a highly personal decision. No two people's reasons, attitudes, and feelings are exactly alike and no one should enforce his views on another.

AFTER A POSITIVE TEST RESULT:

- LET HIM FEEL WHATEVER HE'S FEELING. Don't argue, even with good intentions, that his fears are inappropriate or exaggerated.

- ENCOURAGE HIM TO THINK IT THROUGH for a few days before taking action of any kind. No matter what the situation is, a few days won't make much difference. If he's troubled, you might help best by finding the phone number of an experienced counselor. A second, confirming test is always a good first step.

- DON'T INSIST ON CONFRONTING DENIAL, if that's what he chooses. Some people experience a degree of shock over the test and aren't capable of dealing with the situation immediately. Bring up the discussion again later after the initial shock wears off.

- REASSURE HIM OF YOUR CONTINUED SUPPORT. Whatever comes up, you'll be there to help in any way you can—just as hundreds of thousands of gay men and lesbians have already helped one another.

AFTER A NEGATIVE TEST RESULT:

- Celebrate, if that's what he wants. Now he needs support to stay uninfected. A good discussion of future sexual plans might be appropriate, as well as periodic retesting (a single negative test result is not enough, since it can take as long a year after contact for some people to show detectable antibodies in the test).

Coping with a Diagnosis of ARC

The vague clinical category often referred to as ARC or lymphadenopathy syndrome (LAS) suggests that infection with the virus has progressed to some degree and that the person's immune system is weakened. The hallmark of this condition is *uncertainty* and a string of new questions: *"What does it mean?" "What can I expect?" "What should I do?"* Unfortunately, no one has any absolute answers to these questions. The situation is further complicated when we experience fatigue and malaise as symptoms, as these are very difficult to distinguish from depression. When diagnosed with ARC we have the added and confounding burden that we are not given the special recognition and understanding typically given to friends with full-blown AIDS. Instead, we wonder to ourselves *"Am I really that sick, or am I just being lazy?" "Is it a physical or mental problem?"* People with ARC have sometimes reported a surprising sense of relief upon getting a full AIDS diagnosis, saying *"Now at least I know what's really wrong."*

As a person with ARC or a friend to one, we must understand this uncertainty. The concerns and fears must not be minimized, nor should they be overly encouraged. Friends must:

- GIVE REASSURANCE OF SUPPORT (within reasonable limits); be there for each other in whatever ways the friendship calls for. Sometimes, this just means being a good companion.

- SUPPORT HEALTH-PROMOTING ACTIVITIES, such as increased attention to rest, nutrition, and exercise.

- DISCOURAGE HEALTH-DAMAGING ACTIVITIES, such as drug and alcohol use. Sometimes, the least invasive way to discourage them is simply not to take part in or support them.

- ACCEPT EACH OTHER'S FEELINGS, whatever they be.

It is in this stage of the illness that people are most likely to begin involvement with support groups of one form or another. While such groups can help in very important ways, they can also add stress to existing relationships. Does reliance, even intimacy, with the group somehow suggest that needs aren't being met by the friend or lover? Does one person feel left out of an important aspect of his friend or lover's life at this critical time? Will newer, perhaps more sensitive, or more attractive, friends come on the scene to the diminishment of the existing relationship? Certainly, these are not unexpected fears. Both people should openly discuss their feelings about group involvement. Communication is the key to preventing this type of problem. With it, the partner who feels threatened or somehow minimized can get the reassurance he needs. In many cases, friends and lovers of people who are ill find help in groups of their own, such as those aimed at the "worried well."

Coping with a Diagnosis of AIDS

Most people with AIDS survive for more than a year after their diagnosis. A surprising number are still living five years after their diagnosis. Many couples and loving friends experience a honeymoon period shortly after the diagnosis. They see friends and lovers with new eyes, with new respect for the value of the relationships. Some even begin to exclude others from their innermost circle, reminiscent of the earliest stages of a relationship. Gradually, as the reality sinks in and the implications are realized, new feelings may arise. Old strains in a relationship may surface once again, yet the bond of love often remains stronger and more deeply appreciated.

Individual partners in a relationship may adapt to the reality of the illness at differing rates. Debates can arise over the proper medical or spiritual approach to the disease. People also vary in how they choose to deal with their feelings. For some, denial is an important coping mechanism, while other are more comfortable talking about their feelings. Conflicts may ensue. At times the well partner may feel at a disadvantage. As one man put, *"How can you get angry at someone who is sick and may die?"*

Altogether, an AIDS diagnosis typically presents one of the greatest challenges any relationship may face. To get the most from the relationship, under the most trying of times, a few suggestions:

- LET THE PERSON WITH AIDS CARRY AS MANY OF HIS OWN BURDENS AS HE WISHES. Being made to feel helpless and dependent, even if done out of love, is demoralizing.

- FIND THE DESIRED BALANCE BETWEEN OFFERING AND ASKING FOR HELP. No two people are alike in this regard. Some find it very hard to ask for help, and prefer that others be sensitive enough to offer it. Others would rather tell people when they want help. Communication is the answer, and it can be very direct on this matter: *"How do you think we should handle it?"*

- LET EACH PERSON'S LIFE HAVE IT'S OWN PURPOSE, SATISFACTIONS, AND MEANING. They weren't the same before one became ill, and it's okay if they're not the same now. If the one who is ill chooses not to fight endlessly, he should be allowed his choice, no matter what loss a healthy friend may feel.

- DON'T DWELL ON THE LIKELIHOOD OF DYING, BUT ON THE QUALITY OF LIVING. Unless it's his choice, the person who is ill doesn't need to be engaged in an endless medical discussion. Find as many things to do and talk about as possible which don't revolve around AIDS. Give yourselves a day off.

(For those with AIDS)
- BE CLEAR AND DIRECT WITH FRIENDS ABOUT WHAT YOU WANT FROM THEM, AND WHAT YOU DON'T WANT. Friends who aren't ill, or who don't have full-blown AIDS, may never fully appreciate what the person with AIDS is going through, so don't expect them to anticipate your wishes.

(For those who are well)
- DON'T IGNORE YOUR OWN FEELINGS AND NEEDS. You can't help an ill friend if you aren't whole yourself. You needn't submerge your own feelings and fears, needn't be abused in any way, and needn't lose your own identity. You offer a friend the most when you are full of life and in touch with yourself.

In a relationship stressed by AIDS, perhaps the most important rule is to keep the lines of communication open, both between each other and within ourselves. Keep listening, keep learning, and keep loving.

Coping with the Final Days and Loss of a Loved One

For many AIDS patients, there is a long period in which hope is appropriate. Every reasonable avenue can be explored as science gains knowledge and experience with treatment. With each year, the life expectancy of AIDS patients is increasing. Currently, though, even the best of treatment options is only a stopgap measure which helps us hold on until the next development. At some point in the course of the disease, however, physical deterioration can reach a point of no return. Additional time, if possible at all, may come only with greatly added pain and loss of quality of life.

Our lover or friend is dying. The patient knows it and comes to accept it. Similarly, loved ones and friends must go through a process of letting go of the final hope and attachment. For some, a calm serenity surrounds the relationship, old conflicts are forever forgotten and forgiven. In the best of situations, there is a coming together of close friends, family, and lovers, at peace with each other and the inevitable. It is a profound and moving scene, one which is engraved indelibly on the memories of all who have experienced it. As the time comes closer, less energy need to be expended fighting disease—the doctor will provide medication primarily to relieve pain. All that is required is our presence and love. Mutual loving support may extend outward to others involved in our loved one's care. In a sense, this can be one way in which our friend lives on beyond his death. The love within him, at the final moment, seems released and shared fully among ones who loved him.

It is not always this peaceful, this beautiful. Some, especially those who are taken quickly without time to understand and accept, meet death with fear and rage, and place unreasonable demands on the people around them. When we encounter such a moment, we are forced to confront deep emotions in the harshest of ways. We must forgive the fear and anxiety which made the moment so difficult. For many, this is an appropriate and very important time to seek guidance from the many services available to us.

In a society which does not acknowledge the deep connection that gay people can have with one another, the impact of mourning the loss of a close friend or lover often gets overlooked. Extra care is needed, and it must come from each other. Employers must come to understand that typical work efficiency cannot be expected of us at these moments, any more than it can when a heterosexual worker loses a spouse or family member. This may be a challenge for many employers, especially if it's the fifth such loss experienced by the same worker this year. It's hard for outsiders to comprehend the magnitude of the losses we are suffering. As friends, we must be willing to set aside our agendas, however important, to provide unqualified support to each other. Once we can no longer experience our suffering at the loss of a loved one, we have lost the capacity to be fully alive. To the extent that we can continue to mourn our dead, we have survived the Age of AIDS.

STEP FOUR: IMPLEMENTING THE PLAN

It is important for each of us to know that we whatever challenges we face, we need not face them alone. The support of friendship among us is backed up by the remarkable resources of our community. Community volunteers, health care professionals, paid and volunteer counselors, hotline services, food and financial assistance, information and referrals—all are available for the cost of a phone call. The gay community, particularly in the larger urban areas, offers outstanding services for assisting persons with AIDS and their loved ones (see the *Resources Appendix* of this book for more information).

Putting a personal plan of action in place requires that (1) we set mileposts to remind ourselves that we're moving toward a goal, and (2) we establish a system of personal consequences and rewards to move us along the way. In Step One, we examined our social situation, looking for things we'd like to change. In Step Two, we set goals for making these changes. In Step Three, we described action steps for getting where we want to go, and listed the resources we will make use of. All that's left is the doing. With the help and support which has grown up in this remarkable community, there's little reason not to reach our goals.

Step 4: Implementation

Instructions:

In this last step, list 2 things: (1) any mileposts along the way you might use to measure progress toward your goals (such as an increased number of friends, etc.), and (2) any rewards or consequences you might set for yourself as an incentive. Since improvements in your social life are so rewarding in themselves, you might only think of how best to indulge yourself in newfound resources.

GOAL #1: Mileposts _____

_____

Rewards/consequences _____

_____

_____

GOAL #2: Mileposts _____

_____

Rewards/consequences _____

_____

_____

GOAL #3: Mileposts _____

_____

Rewards/consequences _____

_____

_____

CHAPTER

EXERCISE AND NUTRITION

PART ONE: EXERCISE One of the most common and destructive stereotypes of gay men is that we are physically weak. Unfortunately, many of us have internalized this message and have come to see ourselves as such. Reality, however, is much to the contrary. The truth is that strength and courage have long been a hallmark of our community. As so many of us experienced as children, nothing builds strength and courage faster than being singled out as "different."

Throughout history, gay people have been widely associated with athletic competition, body building, and numerous health movements. Homophobic influences and our own fears of discovery have often worked hard to hide this fact.

Until recently, our involvement in athletics and the fitness movement was often motivated by generalized health concerns and a legitimate interest in looking our best. Gayness celebrates the beauty and attractiveness of the male body, so many of us have sought to make the best of what nature has given us.

Recent research, however, suggests that exercise and fitness may play an even more important role. Studies now show that the activity of

T cells and B cells produced by the immune system is enhanced through exercise. The mechanism by which this occurs is related to the production of pain-killing chemicals in the brain, called endorphins. Exercise stimulates production of endorphins, which in turn enhance the activity of T and B cells. This process is so well-defined that some AIDS treatment research is being conducted with drugs which regulate the production of endorphins.

Before getting into specifics, it's critical to understand that exercise alone cannot make anyone completely safe. Nor will it in any way "cure" those who are already ill. The image of health projected by a firm build or strong body must not be mistaken for health itself. Exercise and fitness must be part of a comprehensive strategy—not a substitute for one.

Developing a balanced, personal perspective about where exercise and fitness fit into your overall strategy is a good place to start. Most importantly, we need to examine how exercise and fitness efforts relate to the two key aspects of facing AIDS: (1) *minimizing the risk of exposure to the virus,* and (2) *strengthening our body's defenses.* Exercise can help or hurt on both counts.

MINIMIZING THE RISK OF EXPOSURE:

How Exercise Can Help	How Over-emphasis Can Hurt
Increased involvement in health-conscious activities.	Builds false security based on appearances, overlooks prevention.
Increased association and social involvement with other men who are concerned about health.	Excess concern over appearances, sometimes leading to the use of immuno-suppressive steroid drugs and shared needles.
Increased self-confidence, sexual attractiveness and opportunities (helpful if it includes a commitment to safe practices).	Increased self-confidence, sexual attractiveness and opportunities can lead to unsafe practices.

STRENGTHENING OUR BODY'S DEFENSES:

How Exercise Can Help	How Over-emphasis Can Hurt
Increased T and B cell activity.	Depleting energy reserves.
Strong motivator in an overall health plan; visible rewards build commitment.	Obsessive behavior to the exclusion of other activities.
Often encourages improved attention to nutritional practices.	Unbalanced fad diets, nutritional deprivation, serious weight loss.
Social involvement in a healthy environment provides support for other health goals, such as quitting smoking or reducing alcohol or drug use.	Social pressure may lead to diminished concern over harmful practices, such as the use of immuno-suppressive steroids.

Direct and Indirect Benefits of Exercise

Establishing and maintaining a regular, well-balanced exercise routine can be an important part of your Integrated Health Plan. In addition to the benefits directly provided by exercise, indirect benefits are often derived as well:

- IMPROVEMENTS IN APPEARANCE

- REDUCED MUSCULAR TENSION

- AN OUTLET FOR STRESS AND FRUSTRATION

- RELIEF FROM DEPRESSION, INCREASED ENERGY

- SOCIAL CONTACT IN HEALTHY ATMOSPHERE

- IMPROVED SLEEP

And, if we exercise at the gym, it allows us to spend time with hot, sweaty, firmly-muscled men in various stages of undress.

Being fit allows us to live, work, and play more easily. Exercise can be a source of healthy social activity and provides opportunities to make new friends.

Group support can make exercise more productive and can be a big help in intervention programs, such as quitting smoking or breaking other addictions. In addition to the direct physical benefits provided, all of these can help you feel better about yourself. It's not just biochemistry that makes a *fit body* the best *antibody*.

WHAT IS FITNESS?

Does "fitness" require a massive chest and a tight, rippled stomach? Bulging biceps, firm thighs? While those sound good (actually, they sound GREAT), they are not a good measure of fitness. A stocky body builder might be less fit than a trim dancer, swimmer, or drag queen. Gay people come in all shapes and sizes and often have personal preferences about their body images. All can be fit, despite wide differences in appearance. Technically, fitness means above-average performance on several measures of physical health, mainly *cardiovascular fitness* (endurance, stamina), *strength*, and *flexibility*.

Arthur Steinhaus, a noted research physiologist, suggested that we are "fit" when we have *"heart, lungs, and muscles adequate enough to handle easily the tasks each day brings."* In other words, FITNESS IS A PERSONAL MEASURE, not an absolute one. At its most basic level, fitness is the ability to comfortably manage our daily routine and have enough energy and drive left over to meet emergencies and enjoy leisure activities.

Cardiovascular Fitness

Dr. Kenneth Cooper has been responsible for popularizing another term for cardiovascular fitness—"aerobic power." Both phrases describe:

> . . . *the ability of the heart, lungs, and circulatory system to provide nutrients needed by body cells to perform work for extended periods of time.*

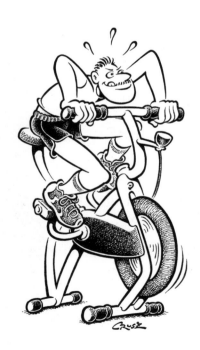

Aerobic or "air-using" activities and exercises improve the efficiency of the heart and thereby improve the flow of oxygen through the bloodstream to the working muscles. The heart pumps blood to the lungs, where the blood picks up oxygen; the oxygen is then delivered via the bloodstream to the various body tissues.

When our heart, lungs and circulatory system become less efficient at transporting oxygen throughout the body, we experience the result as diminished capacity. In other words, we tire easily, can't run as far or as fast, can't work as much without becoming exhausted. Many believe this type of generalized weakness probably extends to all body functions, including the immune response, since nearly all are at least indirectly dependent on a good supply of oxygen. We often think of blood as our lifeline, but it is so only because it carries oxygen to all our cells. It is the oxygen which makes things work.

One of the best known and most accurate measurements of cardiovascular or aerobic endurance is called maximum oxygen uptake, or "VO^2 max." This refers to maximum amount of oxygen the body can use in a minute. This "VO^2 max" is commonly tested using a tread-mill or bicycle-like device. The treadmill is connected to electronic devices which measure the effort being expended, while another device collects exhaled gases for analysis. Rigorous exercise continues for a specific period of time while the electronic hardware measures what's happening to your body.

Fortunately, a low-tech test is also available, one which you can administer yourself. Using it, you can test your endurance by checking your pulse after a predetermined amount of exercise. The pulse is then taken several times, measuring how long it takes before it returns to normal. Shortly, instructions will be provided for performing such a test on your own to assess your cardiovascular fitness.

Strength

Many gay men have discovered firsthand that muscular development can be achieved without excessive effort. The attractiveness of a well-toned male body provides all the motivation that's needed. Because strong bodies look good (read: sexy), and feel so nice, many gay men have done a worthy job in building strength. It hasn't been entirely cosmetic; those biceps are for real. STRENGTH is also the component of fitness most directly associated with our attitudes of self-confidence and competence.

Every movement we make involves muscle action and thus requires strength. Strength and muscle tone aren't only for lifting weights and looking good. Poor muscle tone, for example, is a principal cause of strains and pulled muscles, including chronic lower back pain.

For our purposes, strength may be defined as *the ability to exert force to overcome a resistance* (for example, lifting a weight).

A muscle is simply a mass of fibers. The more muscle fibers that can be involved, the greater the force they can exert when working together. In that sense, it's a lot like community action. There are two common ways to increase strength.

1. *By gradually and progressively increasing the amount of resistance* we try to overcome, we train the muscle to work more efficiently and use more available muscle fibers. This process builds endurance and is described as improving the muscle tone.

   Using relatively light weights or resistance for a large number of repetitions promotes endurance, or muscle tone. Using this approach, we can gain strength without increasing muscle mass or getting any bulkier. Many fitness professionals recommend this rather than continually building more muscle fiber.

2. *By progressively lifting heavier weights a fewer number of times,* we can force muscles to become stronger. This is useful for building muscle mass. The presence of the sharp, tearing pain so prized by the *"no pain, no gain"* crowd is a sign that you are building mass rather than toning.

Both approaches are important to fitness and preventing injuries. The choice of one over the other must be based on your individual situation. If you've always been thin and have little muscle mass, you might want to build muscle mass. If you already have adequate bulk, toning might be more important. Building excessive muscle mass can lead to future problems and may require a lifetime commitment to toning to avoid the "chunky" look that comes with age.

The primary methods we use to build strength all involve some form of "overcoming resistance." We overcome resistance when we lift weight, when we we run, pushing our weight against gravity, or when we pull against the cams and levers of exercise machines. In a similar way, overcoming these forms of physical resistance help us gain the confidence to overcome other types of resistance as well. We learn to face new challenges, on our own and as a community. We learn of our own strength as individuals and collectively as a community.

Flexibility

As David showed Goliath, as Ninja showed Sumo, and as we all know in the bedroom, there's more to life than strength and lung capacity. As we grow older, FLEXIBILITY becomes increasingly important. Research has consistently shown that sedentary or inactive people experience a number of unpleasant limitations:

• REDUCED RANGE OF MOTION in the joints, pain

• LOSS OF ELASTICITY in working muscles, resulting in reduced capacity and early muscle fatigue

• GENERAL MUSCULAR TENSION in key postural muscle groups, resulting in poor posture, stooping, chronic back pain

Some people believe that stiff, less flexible bodies are a storehouse for stress and emotional tension as well. The soothing effect of a good massage would seem to support this view. A variety of stretching exercises can reverse this tendency to rigidity and restore movement to stiff joints. Every fitness program should include static stretches to relax muscles before and after endurance or strength training activities. Yoga is a well known example of an activity that can improve flexibility, and even build muscle tone in specific areas.

A fitness program which fails to address flexibility is likely to create problems that wouldn't have occurred otherwise. Fitness without flexibility is a lot like a self-development program which teaches self-confidence and assertiveness, yet ignores sensitivity. The student might learn to believe in and to speak up for himself, but if he is insensitive to the needs of others, he is invariably headed for abrasive relations. Likewise, a fitness program without attention to flexibility will result in a body system in conflict with itself.

PSYCHOLOGICAL IMPACT OF FITNESS

The community's interest in fitness is a particularly healthy development for gay people from a psychological, as well as physical, point of view. Many of us can recall childhood and adolescent experiences to the contrary. Do any of these ring a bell for you?

• being the last one chosen for teams;

• forced participation in gym activities, often accompanied by the taunts of our peers (swimming and wrestling were fun, though, once you got into them);

• exclusion from sports because of other interests which labelled us as "different" (such as music, art, academics, crocheting, Hollywood hero worship, couch-potato practice, etc.);

• endless references to the supposed weakness of the "sissies" and "fags," a group we knew somehow included ourselves.

Despite obvious side benefits (remember the locker and shower rooms?) these experiences often led us to harbor negative feelings about our physical strength, self-image, and masculinity. Today, such events as the Annual Gay Games provide many with an opportunity to participate and develop skills through training, while giving others a more accurate picture of gay athletics and fitness. The fitness craze which has swept the country in general, and our community in particular, has helped instill in us a new and legitimately proud outlook on our bodies and our identity as gay people.

Balanced Fitness Planning

Fitness in the truest sense encompasses all of these elements—cardio-vascular, strength, and flexibility—and body composition as well. The National Institutes of Health (NIH) estimates that 34-million Americans endanger their health by exceeding their desirable weight by 20% or more. Some fat is necessary on every body and heredity is thought to be a factor in determining one's weight. It is possible, however, to control excess weight by adherence to a balanced diet and a healthy level of physical activity.

Appearance alone will not tell whether a person is physically fit. A slim, highly active dancer who never works out in a formal sense may be in better condition, especially in cardiovascular endurance, than the devoted iron pumper with the sharply defined chest (sigh...). We must avoid defining our fitness by any single activity. Variety is not only the spice of life; in this case, it's the staple, the basic commodity. Besides, getting into shape should be fun and will produce results faster if it's enjoyable. As long as the activities are well-balanced among the components of fitness, we can improve our endurance, strength, and flexibility considerably while having a good time.

The common adage, *"no pain, no gain,"* is a poor guide for evaluating fitness efforts. Instead, we need to select a *balanced* series of activities we enjoy and can live with. If we hate the program we've chosen, there is little likelihood we'll remain committed to it.

Exercise as a Social Activity

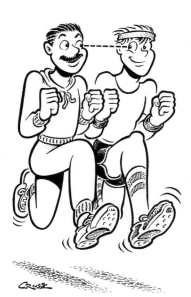

Making exercise a part of our overall health plan can have social as well as physical benefits. Working with an exercise partner can help overcome the sense of boredom which sometimes accompanies repetitious activities and can be a good way for couples to spend time together in a relaxing atmosphere. Of course, it can also bring people to blows over who's cruising or getting cruised by whom.

Community activities which focus on exercise can provide opportunities to meet new people in a non-threatening environment. A few fitness activities which lend themselves to social involvement:

JOGGING	BICYCLING
HIKING	SWIMMING
WINDSURFING	DANCING
WRESTLING	TEAM SPORTS
AEROBICS	WALKING

Dance halls where people can exercise to music have long been a part of our culture. Health concerns seem to have hurt the business at some dance bars, but this is unnecessary. Dance bars never harmed anyone. When there has been a problem, it's been our own extremes of self-indulgence at fault. Dance bars have served many good purposes for us, providing such benefits as:

- companionship

- cardiovascular and endurance exercise

- opportunities to meet (or look at) new people

Fear of AIDS doesn't require that we give up good times at our clubs. "Hot and sweaty" still has a place in our vocabulary. We should be perfectly capable of enjoying ourselves without excess use of alcohol and drugs or careless sexual expression.

Wherever we do it, however we do it, exercise can easily be integrated into our lifestyles. Not having the money to join the latest health spa is no excuse for a sedentary lifestyle.

**STEP 1
WHERE AM I NOW?**

Before embarking on a fitness plan, we need to take stock of our current condition. Some people are already getting the maximum benefit from fitness efforts, while others are leading very sedentary lifestyles which deprive them of possible benefits. Some may even be overdoing it, stressing their bodies unreasonably in pursuit of the perfect build. Starting from an an honest perspective helps resist our social pressures to overindulge and/or under-exercise. It's also useful as a basis for setting realistic expectations.

A second valuable aspect of self-assessment is a subjective evaluation of your physical body image. Do you feel you are too heavy, too thin, or just right? Also, is the weight distributed the way you like? There are few absolutes in this regard, so what matters most is our own perception and preferences.

Finally, it's important to realize that all movement, because it involves muscles, is an exercise of sorts. In that sense, all of us are already involved in some form of fitness activity. We are by no means limited to jogging, calisthenics, or heavy workouts as a means of exercising. Describe whatever form of activity your are currently involved in on the PHYSICAL ACTIVITY INDEX on the following pages.

Physical Activity Index

Instructions, Part One:

Describe the most demanding physical activity you engage in on a regular basis. This will be called your PRIMARY FITNESS ACTIVITY. It might be such things as a workout at the gym, jogging, swimming, walking to work, *serious* shopping, etc.

MY PRIMARY FITNESS ACTIVITY: _____

Next, RATE THE INTENSITY of the activity on the scale provided. Then RATE THE DURATION (how long the activity typically goes on) and RATE THE FREQUENCY of the activity (how often you do it). Circle the number in each column which best describes your activity.

INTENSITY SCORE (circle one):

5 = Sustained heavy breathing and perspiration, as in long-distance running or seriously competitive sports

4 = Intermittent heavy breathing and perspiration, as in tennis or moderately competitive sports

3 = Moderately heavy, as in cycling or recreational sports

2 = Moderate, as in sports such as volleyball, softball

1 = Light, as in fishing or gentle walking

DURATION SCORE:

4 = Over 30 minutes
3 = 20 to 30 minutes
2 = 10 to 20 minutes
1 = Under 10 minutes

FREQUENCY SCORE:

5 = Daily or almost daily
4 = 3 to 5 times a week
3 = 1 to 2 times a week
2 = Few times a month
1 = Less than once a month

Now CALCULATE YOUR TOTAL ACTIVITY SCORE using the following formula: multiply your score for each category times the others.

INTENSITY □ times DURATION □ times FREQUENCY □ = TOTAL ACTIVITY □

EVALUATION OF ACTIVITY SCORE:

Compare your TOTAL ACTIVITY SCORE to the scale below to see where you stand as compared to average.

SCORE	EVALUATION	ACTIVITY LEVEL
100	Very active	Very High
60 to 80	Active and healthy	High
40 to 60	Acceptable, average (room for improvement)	Fair
20 to 40	Below average (inadequate for a healthy person)	Poor
Under 20	Sedentary (will lead to problems for otherwise healthy person)	Very Poor

Instructions, Part Two:

Check the box(es) which best describe how you feel about your physical image.

☐ Don't ask!　　☐ Too heavy　　☐ Too thin　　☐ Just right

☐ A little too heavy　　　　☐ A little too thin

☐ Weight about right, need to redistribute

☐ Satisfied, but need to be more active

Implications of the Activity Index

The activity categories and evaluations described in the previous exercise are only a general guide, not an absolute measure of health. They are meant to apply to people who are in otherwise good health. If you are ill with AIDS or ARC, the significance of these evaluations might be entirely different. For example, a below average or somewhat inactive lifestyle might be appropriate and necessary for someone recovering from a bout of pneumocystis. The value of rest and lowered activity levels is debated frequently by researchers; it's safe to say that no one has the final answer.

The level of activity which is appropriate for your individual condition should be determined through discussion with your physician. Almost all will agree, however, that we all need some degree of activity to remain healthy and make the best of whatever physical capabilities we have.

Determining Fitness Levels

Now that you've evaluated your ACTIVITY SCORE using the PHYSICAL ACTIVITY INDEX and described how you feel about your body image, you can further determine WHERE YOU ARE by testing yourself on the components of physical fitness described previously. If you wish, you can stop reading at this point and perform the tests which follow. Or, if you prefer, you can continue reading and perform them at a more convenient time. If you're reading in the subway on the way home from work, you would probably cause a bit of a stir by taking the tests now (at least in some cities). New Yorkers and San Franciscans, however, are encouraged to do what comes naturally, as the local audience just might appreciate it.

In less than 15 minutes, the simple tests which follow can help you evaluate your fitness relative to other people your own age. Dress in light or loose, comfortable clothes. You'll need a clock, tape measure, and a sturdy chair. Since these same tests have been taken by thousands of others, you can compare your scores with theirs. Be honest with yourself and don't strain beyond your capacity just to make a high score. Whether you score the lowest on record, or higher than Arnold Schwarzenegger, no one else will know. On average, only two out of every hundred people who take these tests achieve "excellent" scores, and only about a dozen rate "good."

Look at it this way—the more out of shape you are now, the easier it will be to improve your score. Whatever your score, think of it as establishing a baseline, a point from which things will only get better.

To make it more interesting, try to get a friend, a roommate, a date, or your lover to take the tests with you. Joint involvement can add to your motivation and make it easier to finish what you start. And if working up a sweat stimulates other interests, there's little reason not to pursue them. Safely, of course.

As a follow-up, you might meet with that same person again in about 3 months and compare progress. Feel free to make a game of it, but try to avoid being overly competitive. In the end, it only really matters to you, since you're the one who will feel better when you make progress.

Fitness Assessment

Instructions

CALCULATE YOUR BODY MASS. If you've got one, keep a calculator handy, as it can be useful for working with the figures involved in finding your BODY MASS INDEX. If you're one of those rare people who remembers how to do math without one, the calculator won't be necessary. Follow these steps:

A. Weigh yourself nude (see—we told you it would be more fun with a friend). If you're feeling modest, subtract a few pounds to account for whatever clothes you choose to wear. Then convert your weight to KILOGRAMS by dividing by 2.2, rounding off the result.

Example: If your WEIGHT is 175 lbs., divide by 2.2, resulting in 79.54 kilograms (kg.)

ENTER YOUR WEIGHT HERE: _____ Lbs.

DIVIDE YOUR WEIGHT BY 2.2: _____ / 2.2

= YOUR WEIGHT IN KILOGRAMS: _____ Kg. (called "A")

B. Next, measure your height in inches while standing in your bare feet (no heels, darling). Divide your height in inches by 39.4 to convert to "meters," rounding off the result. Then, multiply the resulting number by itself to equal "square meters" (sq. m.).

Example: If your HEIGHT is 72 inches (6 feet), divide 72 by 39.4, resulting in 1.8274, rounded off to 1.83. Then multiply that number by itself (1.83 x 1.83) resulting in 3.35.

ENTER YOUR HEIGHT HERE: _____ Inches

DIVIDE HEIGHT BY 39.4 = _____ = Your height in meters

MULTIPLY YOUR HEIGHT IN METERS BY ITSELF: _____ = Square of your height in meters (called "B")

C. Finally, calculate your BODY MASS by dividing your WEIGHT IN KILO-GRAMS ("A" from step A) by the SQUARE OF YOUR HEIGHT IN METERS ("B" from step B).

EXAMPLE: If your WEIGHT IN KILOGRAMS ("A") was 79.54, and the SQUARE OF YOUR HEIGHT IN METERS ("B") was 3.35, your BODY MASS is 23.74 (79.54 divided by 3.35).

("A") DIVIDED BY ("B") = _____ = YOUR BODY MASS

D. Now compare YOUR BODY MASS to the BODY MASS INDEX STANDARDS below and decide how you feel about the results.

BODY MASS INDEX STANDARDS FOR MEN

GOOD	under 21
AVERAGE	22-24
FAIR	over 28.5
POOR	over 33

What if your BODY MASS INDEX is lower than the numbers on the scale?

Although not part of the official STANDARDS, a body mass index lower than 18 or 19 might suggest a problem of too little mass, often a factor for people with AIDS or ARC. If your BODY MASS INDEX falls significantly below 20 (for men), you might first recheck your calculations. If they are correct, make a second set of calculations based on your typical weight previous to becoming ill. If your current BODY MASS INDEX is very low, and is quite different from what it was previously, your doctor should be consulted to determine if there is a need for a special diet to rebuild your weight. Do not attempt to correct a problem of this type solely by exercise.

Now check the box(es) below which best describe(s) how you feel about what you've learned in this exercise.

☐ Depressed   ☐ Pleased   ☐ Not surprised

☐ Satisfied the way I am, regardless of the numbers

☐ Anxious for Step Two, committed to improvement

☐ Other? _____

Implications of the Body Mass Index

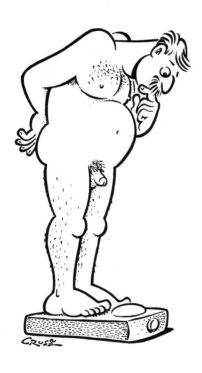

If you aren't pleased with the outcome of the BODY MASS INDEX, it's important not to ignore what it's telling you. When our BODY MASS is higher or lower than it should be, we need to examine numerous related factors, some directly connected, some indirectly.

Excess weight and obesity have well-documented associations with disease. High blood pressure, high blood cholesterol levels, heart disease, diabetes, and certain cancers are far more common in people who are perpetually overweight. While this doesn't deny the fact that people can be "healthy" in spite of less than "average" scores on standard indexes, it clearly suggests that weight and body mass are factors which determine longevity and resistance to certain maladies.

Recently, a myth has arisen that suggests that, since AIDS patients often lose some portion of their weight, an overweight person is somehow "better equipped" to deal with the ravages of the disease. This view, unsupported by evidence, is based on overly simplistic thinking. AIDS creates enormous strains on most body systems, not just on stored fats. Excess weight is sometimes (but not always) a symptom of a sedentary lifestyle and poor nutritional habits. If the major body systems are already overtaxed by excess weight, inactivity, or dietary imbalances, having numerous spare pounds to lose will hardly help in the presence of AIDS or ARC and might well add to the problem.

Aside from the directly physical implications, the worst health risk of excess weight is often psychological suffering—according to the National Institutes of Health. Some (but certainly not all) people who are overweight are unhappy about it. They report that it affects their sexual attractiveness, sexual opportunities, and their self-respect. Some overweight people even report that their career potential is diminished due to common but very unfair prejudices. At the very least, there is little doubt that our psychological outlook has a clear impact on our health.

It's also risky to make too much out of a BODY MASS INDEX rating of "good" or "average." How we score on this index is only one factor which indicates fitness. It's quite possible to look good on this test, yet score very poorly on cardiovascular, strength, and flexibility measures. A true picture of fitness can only be developed by looking at all the indices, not just the one or two which happen to please us.

Yet another set of issues arises for those who fall off the other end of the scale on the BODY MASS INDEX. If our BODY MASS is abnormally low, this too has broad implications.

If low BODY MASS is a result of the disease process of AIDS or ARC, it might signal a need for dietary supplements or diagnostic tests to make sure the body is being properly nourished. It may also be an important factor to consider when setting fitness goals that are realistic and not overly demanding. When a person is unable to retain certain nutrients and store body fats, or when metabolic processes are irregular, potential energy output is almost certainly affected. Pushing the body too hard under such circumstances is dangerous.

For someone unaware of being ill, an unusually low BODY MASS might be a warning sign. If a person has had low BODY MASS for most of his life, there is probably little concern. But when it represents a sudden and recent change, the body may be telling us something very important. Sudden, otherwise unexplained weight losses are one of the most common early warning signs of AIDS and ARC and should be discussed with a physician ASAP.

Regardless of the outcome of the BODY MASS INDEX test, it's important to test our fitness in other ways as well. To do this, continue with the exercises which follow. You may wish to do these now, or continue reading and do them at a later time. Whenever you do them, remember to get down, get sweaty, and get that body in motion. This book, after all, is intended for GAY people.

Cardiovascular Fitness

Instructions:

This test is commonly used for testing the fitness of skiers at the beginning of the season. To take the test, you'll need a common chair (about 17 inches high), a watch or timer, and the ability to take your pulse (at the wrist or neck).

TAKING YOUR PULSE (if you already know how, please skip to THE TEST section):

If you don't know how to take your pulse, here's one method which will work easily with this exercise. Practice it before taking the TEST.

- sit with your arms hanging to your sides

- hold your right elbow loosely against your ribs, bend your right forearm up, pointing it straight out from your body

- turn your hand over so that your palm faces upward (you should resemble Jerry Falwell sitting in a chair facing his flock)

- with your left hand, grasp your right wrist from below (left palm under your right wrist)

- press the tips of your fingers (from the left hand) into the soft area between the wrist bone and cartilage on your right wrist (beneath your thumb); you may need to experiment a bit to find the best spot and the right amount of pressure, but you should now be able to feel your pulse in the tips of your fingers.

There are many other ways to achieve the same result, but be sure to feel for the pulse with your fingers, not your thumb. The thumb has such a strong pulse of its own that it can confuse your count.

THE TEST:

Start when you're rested and comfortable. Have the watch or timer in reach. Stand in front of the chair just as you would before sitting down, with your feet about 3 or 4 inches apart. Then:

- for one full minute, repeat a cycle of sitting down on the chair and standing up again, touching the seat of the chair with your buttocks and keeping your back straight. Do this about once per second, keeping a steady count. If you get bored, imagine yourself moving up and down on... something more enjoyable. Stop at the end of one full minute.

- remain seated on your last cycle and attempt to feel your pulse (no need to count it yet—just find it) ; keep your eye on the time

- at the start of the third minute, count your pulse for exactly 30 seconds

- write the number down and see how it compares to the standards below.

MY SCORE: _____

CARDIOVASCULAR FITNESS STANDARDS FOR MEN

EXCELLENT	35 or less
GOOD	36-44
AVERAGE	45-54
FAIR	55-62
POOR	over 63

Testing Strength

Instructions, Strength Test One — Sit-ups:

One universal measure of strength is the number of sit-ups you can do in one minute, as it is fairly representative of overall strength and endurance. Strength in the abdominal muscles is also important in maintaining good posture, avoiding lower back pain, and is rumored to contribute to sexual endurance.

To do this test, you'll need a watch and either a partner or a piece of furniture to hold your feet down, whichever you find more attractive.

THE TEST:

- Lie down, face up, with your knees bent about 90 degrees; fold your arms across your chest; have your feet securely held down.

- Tuck your chin in toward your chest; while inhaling, bend at the waist and lift your shoulders and torso up until your folded arms touch your legs.

- Exhale while returning your torso all the way to the floor.

- Set your own pace and continue without stopping for one full minute if you can; count each time your arms touch your legs.

- Compare your results to the standards below.

MY SCORE: _____

SIT-UP STANDARDS FOR MEN (NUMBER IN ONE MINUTE)

AGE	14-29	30-39	40-49	50-59	60 +
EXCELLENT	51 +	46 +	41 +	36 +	31 +
GOOD	43-50	35-45	30-40	25-35	20-30
AVERAGE	30-42	25-34	20-29	16-24	13-19
FAIR	20-29	15-24	10-19	8-15	6-12
POOR	0-19	0-14	0-9	0-7	0-5

Instructions, Strength Test Two—Push-ups:

Elbow extensions—push-ups—are commonly used to measure strength in your arms, shoulders, and chest. These muscles help maintain good posture and help us lift and carry weights. Of course, we're all aware of the impression a well-defined chest and firm biceps can make.

THE TEST:

- Lie face down with your legs together, place your hands just outside your shoulders, your fingers pointed forward; keep your back and legs straight.

- Push against the floor, lifting your entire body, until your arms are fully extended; your body should form a flat line and not bend at the joints.

- Complete the cycle by letting your elbows bend until your chest touches the floor.

- Do as many of these as you can in one minute without stopping for rest; remember to breathe rhythmically.

(If it has been awhile since you last exercised regularly or are not at your best for any reason, you can modify this technique by letting your knees remain on the floor. Keep your back and legs in a line and remember to breathe carefully.

- Count and compare your results to the standards below

     MY SCORE: _____

PUSH-UP STANDARDS FOR MEN (NUMBER IN ONE MINUTE)

AGE	14-29	30-39	40-49	50-59	60+
EXCELLENT	51+	46+	41+	36+	31+
GOOD	45-50	35-45	30-39	25-35	20-30
AVERAGE	34-44	25-34	20-29	15-24	10-19
FAIR	20-33	15-24	12-19	8-14	5-9
POOR	0-19	0-14	0-11	0-7	0-4

Testing Flexibility

Instructions, Sit-and-Reach Test

As with STRENGTH, there is no single test which is totally representative. However, lower back muscles and back thigh muscles must remain flexible enough to avoid back pain and leg injuries, so these make a suitable measure of flexibility.

THE TEST:

- Sit flat on the floor near a wall with your legs stretched out; with your shoes and socks off, place your heels against the wall, about 6 inches apart.

- While keeping your legs flat and extended, stretch your arms toward the wall, bringing your forehead toward your knees.

- Stop when you feel a tug in your legs or can't keep your knees flat any longer; hold that position for a few seconds without bouncing or jerking.

- While exhaling and imagining your muscles loosening up, try to stretch a little further; extend your arms toward the wall for about 5 more seconds.

- Check to see how far you've reached, then circle the level below which best describes your results.

SIT-AND-REACH STANDARDS

EXCELLENT	Palms reached flat against the wall
GOOD	Knuckles touched the wall
AVERAGE	Fingertips reached your toes or the wall
FAIR	Fingers came within 1-3 inches of wall or toes
POOR	Fingers remained 4 or more inches from the wall

Implications of the Strength and Flexibility Tests

Having completed these tests, you should have a better picture of WHERE YOU ARE relative to common standards. If you are currently ill with AIDS or ARC, or another disabling illness, remember that the standards don't necessarily apply to you. Depending on your condition, a FAIR or AVERAGE rating might be an excellent score.

If you are not ill, however, and scored poorly against the standards, you may have something to think about. Certainly, there is no need, or desire, for every gay man to be muscular or masculine in the traditional sense. After all, the Stonewall revolution was led by drag queens, not muscle queens. Being fit doesn't require bulging muscles or the "Nautilus" look. What matters is that we take sufficient care of the body so that it at least doesn't add to our problems if illness strikes. A well-cared for and reasonably toned body may be both more resistant to illness in the first place and better able to cope if it occurs.

The conveniences of modern life make it all too easy to under-exercise and over-feed our bodies. The body is a type of machine, with systems built for doing certain types of work. When we don't allow them to do what they're designed for, those systems begin to break down.

Finally, we must acknowledge the link in our gay world between appearance and self-image. Like it or not, gay culture places high value on the appearance of health and fitness. Thus, we owe it to ourselves to make the best of what we've got. If we spend our lives dissatisfied with our physical image, that dissatisfaction almost certainly will have a negative influence on our self-respect and psychological outlook. And that, dearie, has a direct influence on our health.

STEP 2: WHERE DO I WANT TO BE ?

Hopefully, the previous tests have helped you to identify some specific areas you'd like to work on. This might mean improving fitness in one area or another, or simply maintaining the fitness level you presently have. The body operates on a use/disuse principle—

EITHER YOU USE IT OR YOU LOSE IT.

One of our most obvious goals should be to strengthen our natural defenses. We can do that by improving our health and fitness.

Before setting a specific fitness goal, spend a few minutes using the "fitness visualization" exercise on the next page.

Fitness Visualization

Instructions:

Set aside about 15 minutes of uninterrupted time. Turn the phone off, go to the quietest, most comfortable spot in your apartment or home. Dim the lights. Tell the cat to purr.

Begin with the assumption that, over time and with patience and perseverance, you can make major improvements in the way you look or how you feel.

Now begin to visualize an improved picture of yourself, a vision of what you'd like to be and what you'd like to be able to do easily. A few possible thoughts:

- Imagine a strong and fit immune system, strong heart and efficient lungs.

- Imagine a lightness, a gracefulness and agility, associated with improved strength and vitality.

- Imagine the new challenges you will meet and the energy you'll still have after a full day of satisfying accomplishments.

- Imagine how you'll feel knowing your body is at its best, how good you'll feel about yourself and others.

- Imagine the response you'd get (if you want it) from other men, your lover, or that someone you've got your eye on.

Let your mind ponder these images, following them wherever they lead you for about 15 minutes. When you've run out of new ideas, stop and describe the image you saw of yourself in the space below.

_____

_____

_____

_____

Setting Your Goals

Now that you know, in general terms, where you want to be, it's time to get specific—and real—about it. It would be nice to make the changes overnight, but it won't happen that way. Instead, it will occur ONE STEP AT A TIME. In fact, the changes may happen so gradually that your friends might notice them before you do.

That's one reason it's so important to set baseline measures for yourself, so you can see the progress you're making even before it's visible. In STEP ONE, you've already established your baseline measurements. For future reference, you will write them down on the first page of the goal-setting exercise which follows. You may wish to retake the tests again in a month or a few months from now. Regard these initial results as your personal baseline fitness level and take it from there.

Remember not to make your goals so long range that it's too difficult to reach them. Because total physical conditioning is broken down into several components, you may find it easier to target some of the most immediate and specific attributes of getting in shape.

Fitness Goals

Instructions:

First, write down your baseline measurements taken from the PHYSICAL ACTIV-ITY INDEX and FITNESS TESTS you took in STEP ONE.

PHYSICAL ACTIVITY INDEX:	_____
BODY MASS:	_____
SCORE, CARDIOVASCULAR:	_____
SCORE, SIT-UPS:	_____
SCORE, PUSH-UPS:	_____
SCORE, FLEXIBILITY:	_____

Now set goals for the next 9 months which are REALISTIC AND ACHIEVABLE, MEASURABLE AND OBSERVABLE.

	3 months	6 months	9 months
GOAL #1 Weight/Body mass	_____	_____	_____
GOAL #2 Cardiovascular	_____	_____	_____
GOAL #3 Strength	_____	_____	_____
GOAL #4 Flexibility	_____	_____	_____
GOAL #5			
_____ ?	_____	_____	_____

At the end of each period, feel free to review your goals and revise them if you wish. And remember to have fun!

**STEP 3:
HOW AM I GOING TO
GET THERE?**

You'll need to develop a personal exercise program to achieve the goals you've set for yourself. Included here is a general format that you can use in less than an hour, but you may want to tailor it to your particular needs and limitations. You should adapt or substitute any exercise that causes you discomfort. You should begin by doing this routine no more than three times a week and later increase to more often if you wish.

A word of caution about conditioning: because physical changes are gradual and progressive, it's most productive in the long run to start slowly. The soonest you can expect noticeable results is around six weeks. Pushing too hard too soon will increase your chances of hurting yourself and putting yourself through needless agony. You can gradually modify your lifestyle somewhat to become more physically active.

After about 6 weeks, you're likely to hit your first training plateau, during which your performance will level off. It's frustrating and discouraging, but if you hang in there and keep working out, you'll start improving again soon.

To improve your present level of fitness, start out with easy work and give your body a chance to adapt. To make progress, it is only necessary to ask your body to do more than it is used to. This is sometimes referred to as the "overload" principle. Slowly increase the amount of work you do as your body becomes more efficient and capable. Each type of exercise is different, and you're likely to improve at different rates for each.

Each exercise session includes four basic parts:

• WARM-UP

• RESISTANCE WORK

• CARDIOVASCULAR WORK

• COOL DOWN

On the following pages, activities will be described which you can use for each of these. You must, of course, adjust them to your own needs and physical capabilities. After you've read through the suggested activities, use the ACTION PLAN form to describe the actual program you will commit to.

**Warm-up
(5 to 10 minutes)**

The rising of temperature inside the muscles helps prepare you for the rest of the workout and prepares your muscles and joints for the exercise which follows. Walk briskly or walk in place for 3 minutes while you swing your arms at your sides or in wide circles, reach overhead and bend gently side to side; reach arms alternately across your chest with your torso to the left and right, etc.

**Resistance Work
(5 to 10 minutes)**

Either using the weight of your body parts, small hand weights like cans of food or books, or elastic bands, you can do a number of exercises to improve the strength and endurance of muscle groups in your abdomen, arms, and shoulders. Among the standards are the sit-ups and push-ups described in the fitness assessment. Two others are:

SIT-BACKS:
   Starting from a bent-knee, seated position on the floor, fold your arms across your chest and tuck your chin to your chest. Slowly lower your torso back to about a 45-degree angle. Hold until your muscles shake, then return to a sitting position and repeat.

BICEPS CURLS:
   Standing with your feet shoulder-width apart and knees slightly bent, hold your arms outstretched from your shoulders while holding a one-pound can or book in each hand. With your palms facing up, bend your arms at the elbow and bring your hands in until the weights touch your shoulders. Stretch your arms back out to the side and repeat.

For each of these exercises, do the same number of repetitions that you were able to do on the one-minute tests in the fitness assessment, but divide them into 3 sets of one-third to start. Work up to a total of 3 sets of 10 repetitions each. For sit-backs, do as many as sit-ups; for biceps curls, do the same number as on your push-up test.

**Cardiovascular Work
(10 to 30 minutes)**

This is the most important part of any fitness program, since it can help you lose weight and condition your heart and lungs. You should be doing some aerobic exercise at least three times a week for at least twelve minutes and maintain your aerobic fitness. Many popular and fun activities are excellent cardiovascular exercises and you receive benefits from any of them as long as your heart's pumping hard enough. Running is the most obvious mode, but swimming, jumping rope, bicycling, rowing, cross-country skiing, vigorous dancing, and even brisk walking are some others. The intensity and the fact that the activity is continuous are the main points.

Monitoring your pulse is the easiest and most accurate method of knowing whether or not you're pushing hard enough. You can usually locate a strong heartbeat at your wrist or alongside your neck. You want to be exercising at between 70 and 85 percent of your age-adjusted maximum heart rate. This is sometimes called your aerobic threshold or target heart rate range. To find yours, subtract your age in years from 220 and multiply that difference by 70 and 85 percent. Target heart rates are commonly expressed in 10-second figures, so divide each of those one-minute figures by six. This gives you a handy number for counting your pulse during any convenient break in your exercise, and will get you back to work before your pulse starts slowing down again.

Cool Down (5 to 10 minutes)

It's necessary to phase yourself down gently after vigorous exercise to restore more normal circulation and to prevent stiffness and soreness. Cooling down should incorporate some movement and wind up with static stretching.

Walk for at least 2 minutes doing the arm circles, overhead stretches, and arm swings you did when you were warming up. Then spend at least 3 more minutes stretching out, paying special attention to those muscles that received the most strenuous exertion. Include hamstring muscle group stretches to improve low back flexibility, like the following variation on the hurdler stretch.

HAMSTRING STRETCH:
   Sit down as if you were going to take the sit-and-reach test, but place one foot inside against the opposite thigh. Lean gently forward at the waist toward your extended leg and hold that pose. Relax and repeat with your other foot tucked in.

   The sit-and-reach is also a good hamstring stretch.

SHOULDER STRETCH:
   Either sitting or standing, grab your hands together behind your back and slowly raise them until you feel the catchpoint. Hold your arms up without bouncing or jerking.

TRICEPS STRETCH:
   Placing one hand at the top of your spine with your elbow pointed toward the ceiling, reach across and with the other hand, gently pull your arm toward your head.

   Start by doing each stretch once for 5 seconds and build up to doing each stretch 3 times for 15 to 30 seconds each time.

Action Plan

Instructions:

Use the space below, describe your ACTION PLAN for working toward your goals. Consider what you write here to be a commitment you are making to yourself.

TIMES PER WEEK I WILL EXERCISE: _____

PLANNED EXERCISE PERIOD: _____ to _____ (time of day)

☐ (check here for variable time)

DAYS OF THE WEEK (circle)   Sun. Mon. Tue. Wed. Thu. Fri. Sat.

WARM-UP ACTIVITIES: _____

_____

_____

RESISTANCE WORK: _____

_____

_____

CARDIOVASCULAR WORK: _____

_____

_____

COOL DOWN: _____

_____

_____

STEP 4: IMPLEMENTING YOUR PLAN

If you continue working toward your goals, your body will soon respond. Before you begin to see or measure any changes, you may feel the difference in improved energy levels and endurance, or in simply feeling better, less anxious, and more confident about yourself. But in general, the rate of change is so subtle and gradual that you shouldn't depend upon visible virtue being its own reward. After all, getting in shape and staying there is work. It can be frustrating or disappointing along the way, but only persistence will get you there.

In addition to your "action plan" statements to break your goal into smaller steps, you'll probably find it helpful to assign some consequences of real value for succeeding or failing to keep your schedule on track. Many people find it helpful to keep a logbook or diary of your workouts, describing how much, how far, how long they did their exercises. Some people have fun timing themselves during the cardiovascular phase and trying to increase their distance or duration. Be sure to assign yourself a stiff negative consequence for doing fewer than 3 workouts in any week. Some ideas for rewards might include new clothes, especially clothes which emphasize your new "look," sports equipment that you'd really use and enjoy, or even a few personal "indulgences" (safe ones only). Make mutual contracts (not contests!) with your exercise partners or friends at the gym that can even include group incentives like a fitness weekend together skiing or backpacking, or sailing.

Some people find it helpful to post pictures of gorgeous bodies in a visible place to remind them of their goals. Others develop mental images of their idealized appearance to keep the desired results clearly in their minds. At the very least, this type of sustained visualization is a helpful motivator.

Find out what works for you and use it. Share your ideas, insights and experiences with others who are pursuing similar goals. Experiment with ways to build fun and fitness activities into the fabric of your life. Many employers have learned that fitness pays off in increased productivity and reduced absenteeism. Some offer fitness plans, workout facilities, and other assistance for getting in shape. Take advantage of lifestyle discounts on car insurance when possible. If you can't find a group of gay hula-hoopers or whatever, create one.

You don't need a gym or much more than a pair of shorts and a good pair of shoes. If you're exercising at home, even the clothing is optional. The primary ingredient of success is a sincere determination to improve yourself. Beyond that, it's simply a matter of doing it and having fun at it. Go for it!

**PART TWO:
NUTRITION**

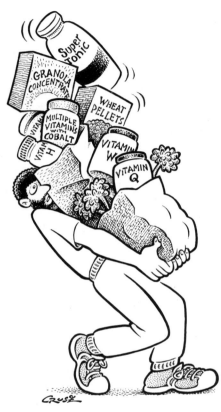

The same growing health consciousness which brings many of us to consider exercise often leads to a review of nutritional practices as well. It makes little sense to try to build up the body through exercise if we don't also take a look at the fuel we feed it. Even aside from its role as a partner to exercise, concern about nutrition has become one of the most common responses to AIDS. There is little question that when the body is under the extreme pressures of AIDS anxiety, ARC, or AIDS itself, a sound diet is fundamental.

Unfortunately, the road to better nutrition is paved with a high-tech blend of good intentions, conflicting claims, and outright snake oil. Perhaps no other aspect of our health care invites as many unsubstantiated claims as nutrition. While the scientific study of the effect of diet on health and illness is relatively new, the sale of magical solutions is as old as mankind. From a purely scientific viewpoint, the interactions of food intake and body process are poorly understood. Only the most extreme problems, such as the link between starvation and disease or certain illnesses and key vitamin or mineral deprivations, are well documented. Yet there is a virtual avalanche of claims directed at consumers about the benefits of diets and nutritional supplements.

The desperation of AIDS has created a ready audience for claims of the curative properties of foods, megavitamins, plants, and special diets. While much of what is offered isn't necessarily harmful, little of it has met even the most rudimentary tests of science. Hardly a week goes by without announcements of new "breakthrough" diets with curative powers, "immune enhancing" substances, or mysterious food supplements. It is equally true, however, that the most traditional health care providers have little training in nutrition. Thus, our most common sources of information often have little more to offer than their own opinions and experiences, based on the limited knowledge of current science.

**A Consumer's
Challenge**

The absence of proven information in the midst of conflicting claims presents a dilemma for many of us. No one wants to miss out on the possible benefits of new discoveries about nutrition, yet most of us can't afford to throw money away, or even risk a fragile balance of health, on unproven remedies. An overall approach must look at nutrition strategies in much the same way as medical therapies, whether "alternative" or "approved." That is:

- CONSIDER THE OPTIONS.
  Learn what's available, both from traditional sources, such as your doctor, and from whatever other sources you wish to consider.

- LOOK BEFORE YOU LEAP.
  Just as you look for real evidence of effectiveness and safety when choosing a medicine, investigate claims made for nutritional products. Ask the tough questions: *What studies have been done to prove what is claimed? How were those studies conducted, and by whom?* (real research is always duplicated and tested by someone other than the people making the claims or selling the product). *What do conflicting sources say about the claims and why? How long have people been using this approach, and what results have they achieved?* (nutrition is as "fad-oriented" as fashion). *What are the possible risks?*

- CONSIDER THE MOTIVES AND QUALIFICATIONS OF THE SUPPLIER.
  Should the claims of a retail salesperson be given the same consideration as those of researchers and career nutritionists? If so, why? In some instances, there might be reason to do so, in others, there might not. While a supplier's impassioned belief might make for convincing salesmanship, it doesn't prove good nutrition.

- MAKE YOUR DECISIONS AFTER CAREFUL REVIEW.
  You might, in the end, decide to try something counter to your doctor's wishes or which sounds too good to be true. But you'll feel a lot better about your choice if it is the result of careful consideration rather than impulse (or the salesman's dreamy blue eyes). Remember, it's your money, and your body. Few of us have the option of replacing either.

There is so much information to sift through on this subject that this book can't possibly do a thorough job. Fortunately, there are dozens of authors writing on all aspects of this subject (see the *Resources Appendix* of this book), and the reader is encouraged to study further before making intuitive leaps. By reading more than one source, we begin to learn the difference between scientific-sounding mumbo jumbo and the real thing. In many situations, the necessary science simply isn't complete and we may need to take action without it. When that is the case, a good rule of safe consumerism is to dismiss out of hand those authors making the most overtly dramatic claims, while listening more carefully to those who admit the limitations of their knowledge.

With these caveats in mind, then, consider the realistic benefits we can expect from proper nutrition:

- *appropriate energy* for physical and mental activities, including exercise;

- *necessary protein, mineral, and vitamin balances* to sustain both normal cell processes and the extraordinary processes of healing;

- *ability to adjust our body mass and image* according to preferences (within the range that is natural to our bodies);

- *ability to store necessary reserves* to combat illness and support our immune responses.

Likewise, consider some of the potential signs and effects of poor nutritional practices:

- *excess body fat,* which contributes to many illness, such as heart disease;

- *emaciation, poor energy reserves,* low capacity for exercise;

- *vitamin and mineral deficiencies* and related illnesses;

- *lowered capacity to fight disease* or tolerate treatment toxicities.

Taking Stock: Nutritional Fitness

Establishing a plan to do something about nutrition begins with taking stock of the current situation. There are two aspects to this regarding nutrition: (1) nutritional fitness (body mass, body image, and energy level); (2) nutritional habits (food selection and eating behaviors). By examining the size and shape of our bodies, we begin to develop an estimate of our nutritional status. While most nutritional disorders in America are due to overeating, weight loss due to HIV infection is a common symptom of AIDS and ARC. Examining and modifying our eating behavior is the only road to better nutrition.

The first consideration in nutritional fitness is the *body mass index* calculated in the *Fitness Assessment* (page 210). It allows us to compare our own body mass to general guidelines. If the results say we have significantly too much or too little mass, it is a good indication that something needs to change. The changes achieved through exercise work best when they are accompanied by reasonable changes in nutritional practices. If overweight is the problem, lowering the amount of fats in our diet will help exercise work off those extra pounds more quickly. Likewise, if our body mass is too low, exercise alone probably won't make it right. Instead, improved dietary intake will be needed to build mass.

The second consideration in nutritional fitness is our *body image,* what we look like. Even though it is a less objective measure than body mass, it plays an important role in our motivation to change eating habits. A quick way to determine body image:

• Strip down (at home, please, not on the bus).

• Standing in front of full length mirror, let it all hang out.

• Look over your shoulder at the rear view; jump around, shake, get things in motion, as you watch carefully.

• Now ask the critical questions: *Does anything jiggle that shouldn't? Which is bigger—chest or waist? Do you like what you see, are you thinner or thicker than you'd like?*

Those who have a history of being overweight may need to check out their perceptions with an honest friend or physician, since they often have distorted body images. The most extreme distortion occurs in anorexia, in which a person perceives himself to be overweight when in fact he is starving. Of course, there are other possibilities, such as people who are too heavy or too thin, but have been that way so long they perceive it as normal. When in doubt, it's best to ask a physician.

The third consideration in nutritional fitness is *energy level.* Body mass and image alone can be deceptive measures of nutritional fitness, especially for younger people. We all know a few people who seem to live on junk food and caffeine, yet somehow still look good (it's so easy when you're young!). Energy level is a highly subjective measure, but each of us knows our own capacities to some extent. To evaluate energy levels, we must compare what we feel at any one time to what we remember to be our natural or regular pattern. Do we have enough *oomph* to get through the day? Does the energy fade as the day wears on? Has it always been this way?

Of course, there are normal variations in energy levels during the day, even for the healthiest of persons. Some recent research seems to suggest that our bodies have a natural longing for the midday siesta common in some cultures. Many factors can influence the amount of energy we perceive:

• activity levels during the day;

• many medical problems, ranging from simple flu and infections to more complex problems such as hepatitis;

- people with AIDS and ARC experience some degree of adrenal failure, which translates directly into listlessness and fatigue;

- psychological conditions, such as depression, mourning, and sadness.

However, when other factors don't account for low energy, it is worthwhile to consider the effect of improper nutrition. Some foods are directly converted into energy in the body. When we don't get what we need, we slow down, much as a flashlight dims when its batteries need charging. One possible source for chronic fatigue (other than illness or anemia) is taking in too few calories or the "empty" calories supplied by junk food. Taking our meals too far apart may also contribute to fluctuating energy levels.

A number of drugs are well known for their ability to stimulate energy levels. Almost all are dangerous, especially for people compromised by illness. Substances such amphetamines, crystal, even the caffeine in coffee and soft drinks, will produce short-term increases in perceived energy, but not in the same way as nutritional intake. Where food actually supplies energy, drugs cause us to use up energy reserves more quickly by putting the adrenal glands in overdrive. For a while we seem invigorated, but there's a price to pay. It's just like overspending on a credit card—the bill will soon come due for living yesterday. This can be extremely damaging for people with AIDS and ARC, regardless of how good it might feel for a few hours. Nutritional intake—food—is the only way to increase energy reserves, just as putting gas in the car is the only way to keep it going.

Nutritional Habits

The second aspect of assessing our current situation is to evaluate our nutritional habits. Food habits can be extremely resistant to change. Although food fads come and go throughout our lives, many of our basic eating patterns were picked up from our parents. Did we learn to greet friends in our home by offering food? Do we prefer fried food or ones with heavy sauces? Is butter a must, margarine a no-no? Is dessert an expected part of every meal? Is meat always the central dish? All of these patterns are likely to have their roots in our childhood, rather than in any conscious process of decision making.

As adults, we are constantly being sold on new habits. The nutritional section is often the largest in bookstores. Food fads and the latest diets, often extolled in books by or for the "beautiful people," promote hundreds of conflicting ways to lose weight. The confusion is only compounded by "experts" who legitimize their opinions with their degrees, each of whom claims to have mastered the one true way to weight control. All the while, traditional science sits back and insists that the only reliable way to lose weight is to eat less. Most research confirms that the weight lost in fad diets tends to return. The weight loss, in fact, may well be due to loss of muscle mass rather than body fat.

A great fallacy of most fad diets is that, somehow, everyone can and should look like (not just at) the slim, tight models used to pitch the diets. The truth is that each of us has an optimal weight, based on such factors as bone structure, body shape, and heredity. For some, this means a stocky build, for others the tall and thin look. No matter how hard we try to be something other than what nature intended, our bodies will continually pull us toward our natural shape. The challenge is to know what that shape is and make sure we neither hang excess fat on it nor eliminate the intended padding. A slow and reasoned approach which permanently changes eating habits is the most effective approach for anyone seeking weight control. This increases the chances of achieving our optimal body weight without depriving us of essential nutrients.

Just as there are drugs which can delude us about energy levels, there are numerous chemical means people use to fight the eating habit. In fact, they are often the same drugs. Drugs which seem to stimulate energy also suppress the appetite. Likewise, most of the drugs which depress the appetite, even non-prescription "dexa-something-or-other" weight-loss pills have a speed-like affect. Hospitals and drug clinics throughout the country treat thousands of people addicted to so-called diet pills, an addiction not unlike that of speed freaks. Whatever the label, whatever the purpose, drugs of this type are highly addictive because of the artificial stimulation they give users. People using them run the risk of nutritional deprivation. Study after study has reported that people who use them for weight reduction inevitably regain any lost weight soon after they stop using the pills.

A balanced, natural approach is all the more important for people with AIDS or ARC. The weight loss so commonly caused by the disease can be harmful in itself if we fail to make up for lost nutrients. Any artificially induced weight loss efforts can be dangerous. When AIDS or ARC, or even an undiagnosed condition includes significant weight loss, special efforts must be made to be sure the body is getting what it needs.

For most people, sound dietary habits have a common foundation:

- eating at least three meals per day, or responding in some way when the body signals hunger;

- eating a balance of fresh foods from each of the major food groups (grains, vegetables/fruit, protein sources) rather than empty calories from junk foods;

- taking in an adequate amount of food, as measured in calories, neither undereating nor overeating to any great degree.

Of course, this is not to say that this is all there is to good nutrition. But it does serve as the foundation or skeleton of a proper nutritional program. Without it, no amount of vitamin or mineral supplements and no magic formulas from a health food store will make up the difference. Dietary supplements must always be used as intended, not as substitutes for natural food sources. The more care we take in getting a nutritional foundation from the freshest, most natural food sources possible, the less need we have for high-priced supplements, pills, and powders.

The most common stumbling blocks to good nutrition include the following:

- *eating only to stop the hunger sensation* (junk foods do this just as effectively as real foods, yet provide little of what we really need).

- *letting excessive work or activity levels override the signals our bodies send us when we need nutrients* (pushing ourselves by will power stimulates excessive adrenalin production—just like drugs—providing higher-perceived energy levels and suppressing hunger signals; hard-driving, "type A" personalities don't need drugs to harm themselves).

- *careless food selection, excessive use of processed or highly prepared foods* (these almost always are nutritionally deficient compared to fresher, more natural foods).

- *dietary imbalances based on personal taste preferences* (a good balance among the food groups is essential, no matter what we like; as adults, we must learn to like the foods we need).

- *high degree of reliance on dietary supplements* (supplements are never 100% effective in making up for dietary deficiencies; while they are helpful in compensating for inherent deficiencies in the typical American diet, their capabilities are limited and they work best in combination with proper food intake).

- *adherence to special diets which rely on large intakes of a very small number of food types* (all-fruit or all-vegetable diets, brown rice diets, etc. ought to be viewed with suspicion; there is virtually no scientific evidence to support their use, and a good deal of evidence to suggest they can be harmful).

Nutrition-Related Diseases

Diet has been implicated in the development of many illnesses, including heart disease, cancer, and diabetes. While it is impossible here to cover each disease in detail, some general recommendations are in order. Diets high in fats (cholesterol) and low in complex carbohydrates have been linked to cardiovascular illness and diabetes. The lack of fiber in the diet has been linked to cancer of the colon and other gastrointestinal disorders. Overuse of salt is suspect of involvement in hypertension (high blood pressure). As a rule of thumb, the purer the food the better. Although the connection is not completely clear, foods which contain a high amount of artificial additives, such as nitrates, have been implicated in some forms of cancer (although it seems like so has everything else).

Natural foods, freshly picked and simply prepared, provide the highest nutritional value and least risk.

Caffeine, a true stimulant, increases the respiration rate, heart rate, blood pressure, and secretion of other stress-related hormones. In moderate amounts (50 to 200 mg per day, or about what we get in two cups of coffee), caffeine seems relatively harmless. Or at least the harm is difficult to measure. Higher amounts can produce reactions in the body that are indistinguishable from those of anxiety attack or amphetamine use. People who drink 8 to 15 cups of coffee daily, for example, may complain of dizziness, agitation, restlessness, recurring headaches, and sleep difficulties. Large amounts of caffeine are also present in tea, colas, chocolate, any many over-the-counter drugs, such as cold remedies and pain killers. Given the stress which we all experience from living in the midst of AIDS, it makes sense to reevaluate our caffeine intake and set reasonable limits. This isn't always easy to do, since long-term use of caffeine results in an addiction-like reaction when we try to cut down.

Based on the previous information, now use the next few pages to evaluate your own nutritional practices.

Nutritional Fitness and Habits

Instructions:

Answer the following questions as best you can.

I.   NUTRITIONAL FITNESS:

1.   What is your *body mass index* (as calculated on page 211), and how does it compare to the guidelines given?

My body mass: _____

Rating according to the guideline: _____

2.   What is your evaluation of your body image (using the brief exercise on page 231)?

☐   Just right

☐   Too heavy for my build
     (how much?)   ☐   a lot   ☐   somewhat ☐   just a bit

☐   Too thin for my build
     (how much)   ☐   a lot   ☐   somewhat ☐   just a bit

3.   How do you feel about your body image (in your own words)?

_____

_____

4.   How would you rate your overall energy levels on a typical day?

        Poor   Average   Very good
         1 ----------- 2 ----------- 3 ----------- 4 ----------- 5

5.   What, if any, causes other than nutrition might be affecting your energy levels (see page 233 for some possibilities)?

_____

II. GENERAL NUTRITIONAL HABITS:

1. How many full meals per day do you normally eat (meals which include foods from two or more food groups)? _____

2. How well-balanced do you feel your diet is?

   Poorly   About average   Very well
   1 ----------- 2 ----------- 3 ----------- 4 ----------- 5

3. Describe your intake of "junk foods" in an typical day:

   1/3 of my diet   Occasional   None at all
   of more   snacks each day
   1 ----------- 2 ----------- 3 ----------- 4 ----------- 5

4. Indicate the degree to which each of the following nutritional practices describes your own habits:

   • *Eating only to stop the hunger sensation*

     Totally me!   Somewhat   Not at all
     1 ----------- 2 ----------- 3 ----------- 4 ----------- 5

   • *Letting excessive work or activity levels override the signals our bodies send us when we need nutrients*

     Totally me!   Somewhat   Not at all
     1 ----------- 2 ----------- 3 ----------- 4 ----------- 5

   • *Careless food selection, such as excessive use of processed or prepared foods*

     Totally me!   Somewhat   Not at all
     1 ----------- 2 ----------- 3 ----------- 4 ----------- 5

   • *Dietary imbalances based on personal taste preferences*

     Totally me!   Somewhat   Not at all
     1 ----------- 2 ----------- 3 ----------- 4 ----------- 5

   • *High degree of reliance on dietary supplements*

     Totally me!   Somewhat   Not at all
     1 ----------- 2 ----------- 3 ----------- 4 ----------- 5

   • *Adherence to special diets which rely on large intakes of a very small number of food types*

     Totally me!   Somewhat   Not at all
     1 ----------- 2 ----------- 3 ----------- 4 ----------- 5

III. SPECIFIC NUTRITIONAL HABITS

Check off the responses which best describe your nutritional habits.

1. I limit the amount of fat and cholesterol I eat, including fat on meats, eggs, butter, cream, shortenings, and organ meats such as liver.

    Always --- Sometimes --- Rarely
    1 ----------- 2 ----------- 3 ----------- 4 ----------- 5

2. I limit the amount of salt I eat by cooking with only small amounts, not adding salt at the table, and avoiding salty snacks (potato chips, pickles, ketchup, hot dogs, cheese, etc.).

    Always --- Sometimes --- Rarely
    1 ----------- 2 ----------- 3 ----------- 4 ----------- 5

3. I make an effort to avoid eating too much sugar, especially snacks such as candy, soft drinks, confections, and ice cream.

    Always --- Sometimes --- Rarely
    1 ----------- 2 ----------- 3 ----------- 4 ----------- 5

4. I make an effort to avoid processed foods, junk foods, and foods with artificial additives (white bread, frozen pizza, TV dinners).

    Always --- Sometimes --- Rarely
    1 ----------- 2 ----------- 3 ----------- 4 ----------- 5

5. I eat regularly planned meals, in a relaxed and pleasant atmosphere.

    Always --- Sometimes --- Rarely
    1 ----------- 2 ----------- 3 ----------- 4 ----------- 5

6. I eat slowly, making sure that I taste each bite and enjoy it.

    Always --- Sometimes --- Rarely
    1 ----------- 2 ----------- 3 ----------- 4 ----------- 5

7. I limit my caloric intake to maintain an optimal body weight and adjust my intake to accommodate changes in my energy output.

    Always --- Sometimes --- Rarely
    1 ----------- 2 ----------- 3 ----------- 4 ----------- 5

8. I limit caffeine intake to less than 200 mg per day (equivalent to two cups of coffee).

      Always   Sometimes   Rarely

        1 ----------- 2 ----------- 3 ----------- 4 ----------- 5

9. I space my meals to avoid states of extreme highs and lows in my blood sugar.

      Always   Sometimes   Rarely

        1 ----------- 2 ----------- 3 ----------- 4 ----------- 5

IV.   CONCLUSIONS

After reviewing all of the above, I would rate my overall nutritional fitness and nutritional habits as follows:

Nutritional fitness (section I:

      Poor   Acceptable   Very good

        1 ---------- 2 ----------- 3 ----------- 4 ---------- 5

Nutritional habits (sections II and III):

      Poor   Acceptable   Very good

        1 ---------- 2 ----------- 3 ----------- 4 ---------- 5

Nutrition and the Immune System

The connection between our nutrition and the immune system is not yet fully understood. Most research examining this issue has studied people in states of serious malnutrition or obesity. These studies show a clear link between these conditions and the rate of infection. It is also known that certain vitamins and minerals play a role in our immunity, at least for people with deficiencies in these substances. No one has proven, however, that using supplements to increase vitamin and mineral levels in basically healthy people in any way prevents disease or enhances immunity. Despite a few claims to the contrary, no one has been able to demonstrate that so-called megavitamin therapies will cure AIDS, and most researchers question whether it has any value at all. There are, however, a few long-living AIDS patients who disagree. It is well-established that excessive vitamin and mineral supplements can actually be toxic, though proponents of such supplements say this can only result from their improper use.

There has long been a long-running scientific debate on the value of vitamin and mineral supplements, with some groups claiming important benefits, even for healthy people, and others insisting there is no evidence to support this. While some scientists, such as Dr. Linus Pauling, have claimed benefits for Vitamin C against colds, other scientists have never been able to duplicate his results. With such lofty scientists in dispute, it is probably beyond any of us to know, or claim, for certain what the role of vitamin supplements may be.

We do know that a well balanced diet has a positive effect on all aspects of health: preventing illness, helping us fight infection, and promoting a sense of well-being. Thus, if our natural diets are deficient in fundamental vitamins—and many processed, preserved, and mass-produced foods are—some degree of vitamin or mineral supplement may be useful. This is a long way from concluding, however, that we should spend all kinds of money on every overpriced pill recommended by the local health food store. There is little or no scientific evidence to support the vast majority of claims made for such products. The manufacturers avoid having to do the research by carefully refusing to make any claims on the product labels, thus preventing action by regulatory agencies. There are no restrictions, however, on what store clerks and self-taught experts say, which more than makes up for the lack of information on the labels. A visit to most such stores will result in a litany of unabashed claims: *"This one is for this. This solves this. This one cures that. This helps stress. This is much better than that, that's why it costs so much more."*

As consumers, we owe it to ourselves to ask:

"Who says so?" or *"Show me the evidence!"*

We need to learn the difference between wishful thinking and sub-stantiated evidence. It would be nice to believe that our problems could be solved by taking pills, but if the magic were there, you would think that someone would take the time and spend to the money to prove it. The fact that manufacturers don't even attempt to do the research is suggestive evidence in itself.

This doesn't prove, of course, that dietary supplements have no value. The point is simply that no one has put much effort into proving it one way or the other. A problem exists only when hyped-up claims are made which go beyond what is actually known. All this is made more important by AIDS, where we are indeed grasping at straws in the absence of proven solutions. It may even be true that people suffering from HIV infection experience greater vitamin and mineral deficiencies and may therefore have a greater need for supplements. But at the very least, those who are ill need to be careful how they spend diminishing financial reserves. The tough questions we ask our doctors about expensive tests and treatments should likewise be asked about every pill, potion, and powder peddled by retail establishments. Sincerity aside, years of working in a health food store doesn't make someone a nutritional expert—only a better salesman.

Special Diets and AIDS

A few clear connections between diet and health, such as the im-muno-suppression caused by stress, invite dietary solutions. For ex-ample, stress seems to result in more rapid depletion of potassium in the blood. Thus, dietary changes which increase the intake of potas-sium-rich foods such as fish, bananas, potatoes, and milk, seem ap-propriate. Whether similar benefits can be attained by taking potas-sium supplements is less-well documented.

Generally speaking, dietary advice for people under stress, or even with AIDS, is the same as that for maintenance of overall health. There are no known diets which have demonstrated, to science's satis-faction, any benefits for AIDS patients. Some, indeed, seem down-right harmful. Diets which promise immune-enhancement or viral cleansing must be evaluated against proven nutritional recommenda-tions. While most doctors may lack special training in nutrition, highly-skilled nutritional specialists are on call at most hospitals. When a special diet asks us to take a radical departure from estab-lished nutritional practices, it must be checked out with a qualified nutritionist, such as a registered dietician.

Changing diets when ill requires special caution and definitely should not be attempted without guidance. For example, switching to a veg-etarian diet demands special care that adequate protein and vitamin intake is maintained. When meat is eliminated from the diet, it is critical that additional sources of protein be used to replace what was formerly taken in from meats. When this care is taken, a vegetarian diet should pose no risks and some possible benefits. Fortunately, vegetarianism is common and well established so people who can guide us in its proper use are easily found.

Some diets, such as macrobiotics, are the source of considerable controversy. While proponents claim special benefits for AIDS patients, doctors and professional nutritionists advise extreme caution. A review of the nutritional components of this diet suggests several important deficiencies. While this may be a matter of personal choice, nutritionists insist that no benefits have been demonstrated for the diet and that there is clear evidence of harm in some instances. Because the dangers of nutritional deficiency are so serious for AIDS patients, thorough research must be done before abandoning a more traditional diet in favor of macrobiotics. This should include discussion of the claims and counter-claims with a physician or certified nutritionist. We may not always choose to believe them, but we should at least hear their views before taking action. The benefits reported by small numbers of people who have been on such diets for relatively short periods, however sincere, are almost certainly subject to the well-known "placebo effect." The real results of a major dietary change, including symptoms of nutritional deficiencies, might take several weeks, even months, to show up.

SETTING A GOAL

We can set nutritional goals for several reasons. (1) After assessing our body mass or image, we have determined that we are over- or underweight. (2) After reading this section, we understand that by selecting and spacing food more carefully we can improve our energy levels and emotional outlook. (3) On the recommendation of a physician or nutritionist, or through our own reading, we have determined a need to change our dietary habits.

For people fighting HIV infection, additional attention to nutrition is particularly important. A common symptom of AIDS and ARC is a loss of appetite. Fevers and infections create an increased metabolic rate and increased need for protein and calorie intake. Poor nutrition may also contribute to further suppression of our immune systems. While optimal nutrition will in no way cure AIDS, it can provide added strength for fighting infections and give us a chance to hold on longer while awaiting a cure.

A person fighting infection may have different nutritional needs from someone who is not ill. An adult man who is not stressed by infection or increased activity levels typically needs about 2700 calories and 56 grams of protein per day. During periods of illness such as AIDS, a man may need up to 5000 calories per day, plus additional protein. Vitamin and mineral supplements may be helpful in moderation.

When appetite is limited due to nausea, diarrhea, or general weakness, it is important that the food we ingest be as nutritious as possible. Nutrient-dense foods, like steaks, peanut butter, fresh vegetables, and pasta provide more nutrition per bite than less-dense goods. Additional fats can be added by using extra butter—something ill advised for most of us—or sour cream. Because of compromised immunity, we should avoid uncooked proteins like raw fish, oysters, and eggs. Meat should be cooked longer than usual and extra care should be taken in food handling and storage to reduce the risk of unwanted bacteria entering our bodies.

For those in advanced stages of disease, good nutrition becomes especially difficult. Shopping becomes a tiresome chore, if possible at all, and growing financial problems make purchasing high quality food all the more challenging. When this is the case, it's time to swallow our pride and ask for HELP. Help is available in abundance from this wonderful community. Friends can do our shopping or can cook large quantities of soup, stews, or spaghetti sauce. Support agencies in many cities provide free food and even prepare meals for those in greatest need—all we need do is ask. Each of us in this situation needs to work out a nutritional plan which includes not only what to eat, but how to get it and how to cook and serve it.

Goal Setting and Action Planning

Instructions:

GOALS:

1. Set a goal for as many of the following aspects of nutrition as you feel necessary:

   ☐ Increase my body weight (by how much? _____   by when? _____)

   ☐ Decrease my body weight (by how much? _____   by when? _____)

   ☐ Improve my energy level (by when? _____)

   (as measured or indicated by _____

   _____)

   ☐ Other goal? _____

   (by when? _____)

   (as measured or indicated by _____

   _____)

ACTION PLAN:

2. Describe the steps you will take to achieve the goals set above. Chose from the suggestions below or add your own.

   ☐ Reduce my risk of health problems from specific foods or seasonings (junk foods? excess salt? cholesterol? fats? preservatives?):

   Specifically, how much and by when? _____

   _____

   _____

   _____

☐ In general, eat more of the following types of foods:

_____

_____

☐ In general, eat less of the following types of foods:

_____

_____

☐ (Decrease) or (Increase) my use of food supplements (vitamins, etc.):

How, why, and by when? _____

_____

_____

_____

☐ Eat at home more often, less often in restaurants

☐ Other changes in my dietary habits?

_____

_____

_____

_____

_____

Implementing the Plan — Feeding the New You

After promoting a skeptical, consumerist view of fad diets and expensive food supplements, it would be difficult for this book to suggest an ideal diet which wouldn't be met with the slings and arrows of those who disagree with this view. There are hundreds of nutritional experts, some real, some poseurs, in every city, just as there are hundreds of books on nutrition. This isn't one of those books, and we thus encourage you to look carefully and more deeply into this subject before setting a brave new course of dietary endeavor.

There are, however, general guidelines that most professionally trained nutritionists seem to agree on. No one would pretend that such guidelines are the final word on nutrition, but they are a valid place to start. Following the guidelines should ensure that we meet our daily requirements for basic nutrition. The plan is meant to be flexible, allowing us to select food we enjoy, rather than forcing steaming seaweed down our unwilling throats. Diets inevitably fail when they ask us to change our food patterns radically and against the advice of our taste buds.

Consider the following loose guidelines and see if they are something you can live with.

DAILY FOOD GUIDE

- 2 servings of low-fat milk products, e.g. yogurt or cottage cheese

- 4 servings of protein foods:

    - 2 servings of animal protein, 3 oz. each (or vegetarian equivalent)—not cooked in oil.

    - 2 servings of legumes (beans, peas, etc.) and/or nuts

- 4 servings of fruits and/or vegetables

    - 1 serving of vitamin C-rich foods, such as oranges, grapefruit, etc.

    - 1 serving of dark green vegetable, such as broccoli or spinach

    - 2 servings of any other fruits and/or vegetables

- 4 servings of whole grain products, such as cereal, bread, and rice

- 1 serving of added fat or oil, such as butter, margarine, oil, etc.

What matters most in the above guidelines is the balance of the various foods. Too much or too little of any of them makes for a poor diet. The freshest, most natural sources will almost always be best, both in taste and in nutritional value. When available, organic foods give the added benefit of being free from potentially harmful preservatives and pesticides. Processed, packaged foods generally are the most nutritionally deficient and are also the most likely to include excessive amounts of salt and other preservatives. Frozen foods can be either good or bad. Frozen raw vegetables can sometimes be more nutritious than the poor quality of produce available in some areas or off-season. On the other hand, processed frozen foods, such as pizzas and TV dinners, typically offer little nutritional value, no matter how appealing they look in their neat little yuppified containers. Getting them to look right in their packaging has more to do with marketing than nutrition. Packaged foods, once the miracle staple of the post war era, are about as good as they look, which isn't saying much.

The cost of truly fine foods is often no higher than the price we're accustomed to paying for packaged marvels of convenience in plastic trays. Changing our diets usually means changing our shopping habits as well, giving substance and value a higher priority than convenience or packaging. Even when high quality foods do cost a little bit more, it is money well spent. Money can also be saved by spending less on sugar water (soft drinks), water with bubbles (name brand bottled water), and chemically treated water (diet drinks).

Making It a Habit

Most of us eat more often than we have sex. Thus, dietary habits are deeply ingrained and changing them can be even more challenging than altering sexual habits. The process, however, is quite similar. It's not enough to say what we won't or shouldn't do. Instead, we must find something appetizing, something tasty, to replace past delights. New habits must conform to generally accepted guidelines about nutrition, and like safe sex, might need a little "spicing up" to live up to our expectations.

Implementing a change in diet requires creativity and care. All the effort spent in careful selection of foods can be wasted in seconds in the kitchen, either by damaging the food through poor cooking techniques or making it so bland as to be unpalatable. Improper cooking of foods can destroy their nutritional value, kill their taste, and burning food may even create harmful chemicals that weren't there when it left the store. Certainly, there is plenty of room for flexibility in cooking styles, and keeping things safe and wholesome is not all that difficult. Fortunately, the most effective cooking methods are often the easiest as well.

FRUITS AND VEGETABLES

Let's face it—Mom was right about vegetables. Both raw and cooked vegetables should be a mainstay of our diet. Even though we may continue eating meat, getting better acquainted with fruits and vegetables can make a big improvement in our diet. Hearty vegetables, such as eggplant, can often take the place of the traditional slab of meat that so long decorated our plates. And then there's zucchini. Who ever said that vegetables weren't sexy?

The money saved by eating in more often can be used to purchase the finest, freshest fruits and vegetables at specialized markets. The local supermarket—bless its little heart—is often too much of a mass production outlet and may not be the best best place to find fresh foods. Most of us need to stop thinking of vegetables only as a side dish and move them center stage. Properly prepared vegetables mixed with rice and a few strategic herbs may be all that's needed for a sturdy and nutritious meal. Asparagus parboiled and chilled makes a great addition to a modern salad. To make new style meals more appealing, learn to pay attention to the food's presentation—combine the right colors, consider the geometric patterns of the dish. Use fruit salads and melon for a colorful snack or dessert, perhaps with a touch of sour cream. Tell your guests that the raspberries you served for dessert (the ones you picked from the bush alongside the road) were imported from New Zealand. It makes them taste better.

Overcooking vegetables destroys many vitamins and minerals and breaks down important proteins. Vegetables are best when eaten raw or cooked only modestly. When properly cooked, they should respond with a degree of crispness or snap when cut or broken—not a soft and soggy *"squish."*

Best cooking methods: *steam cooking, microwave, or quick stir-fry (without a lot of oil; cooking in heavy oils, though tasty, is not recommended).*

PROTEIN

While protein is a mainstay of our diet, most of us have learned to overvalue and overconsume it. Many of our most cherished sources of meat protein, such as steaks and roasts, are marbled with excess fat (that's what makes them so tender and tasty). Lean beef, though, is an excellent source of protein. Sea fish, such as salmon, haddock, and cod, have the added advantage of providing nourishing fish oils which may be beneficial in preventing heart disease. Some nutritionists recommend eating deep-water seafood 3 to 4 times weekly. To avoid adding fats in cooking, learn to use a variety of seasonings to bring out the natural flavors.

Non-meat proteins can be supplied by combining legumes (beans and peas) with complex carbohydrates like rice. Soybean products provide excellent protein and, in creative hands, can be whipped into interesting and delicious dishes.

Cooking meat or fish in oil (frying) adds cholesterol to the diet. Charring or frying to black is suspected of producing carcinogens (possible cancer-causing substances). Undercooking, especially pork and poultry, can lead to food poisoning or parasites.

Bacteria from polluted waters is an increasingly common problem with fish, especially shellfish. It is almost impossible to detect beforehand. A severe illness, *delta hepatitis*, is caused by contaminated shellfish. It is often fatal to people who are carriers of more common forms of hepatitis, and is dangerous to anyone infected with HIV.

Best cooking methods, meats: *broiling (but not blackening), convection ovens, oven baking, and microwave (requires considerable learning to get it right). Special care must be taken when preparing poultry to avoid food poisoning: wash the bird carefully before cooking, cook until no pinkness remains, and, most importantly, wash all cutting boards, knives and utensils, and hands carefully after handling the uncooked bird and before touching anything else (or use separate chopping boards). Bacteria from the birds is commonly spread to other foods, such as salads, by the cook. This, not undercooked poultry, is a major source of food poisoning. Complications of food poisoning are extremely debilitating for those with HIV infection.*

Best cooking methods, fish: *grill, microwave (very easy and very good), oven bake, sauté, or poach; avoid any fish or shellfish which look or smell strange in any way; follow the same guidelines for cleanliness as described above for chicken. Use spices, not oil, to add flavor.*

DAIRY PRODUCTS
As a group, Americans eat far too much dairy food. Milk products should be limited to two portions daily for healthy folks, those wonderfully sexy milk commercials notwithstanding (just who runs that "Milk" association anyway?). Milk, however, is a good source of dense nutrients for those who are ill or having trouble with weight loss. Those without such problems should stick with low fat products—cottage cheese, yogurt, and 2% milk. Tasty desserts can be made with low fat milk and sugar-free custards—save the decadent cheeses, buttery sauces, and ice creams for special occasions. Such occasions should be designated in advance, since, on the spur of the moment, it's all too easy to decide that any moment is "special" when the desserts look good.

FIBER AND GRAINS

Research has shown that the American diet is very often deficient in fiber, the non-digestible part of foods. Vegetables, such as carrots, asparagus, broccoli, and lettuce are particularly good sources, as are hard fruits (doesn't everyone love a hard fruit?), such as apples and pears. Non-refined grains and cereals—whole wheat products, brown rice, bulgar wheat—also fit the bill. Fiber in the diet provides essential cleansing of intestinal tracts and helps keep bowel action regular. This can be particularly important for people who are ill, since many medicines wreak havoc with digestion. When our diets don't contain adequate fiber, we must supplement our natural sources with 2 to 3 tablespoons of prepared fiber each day from sources such as psyllium seeds, millet, and others. Fiber can also be found in coarse breads, such as cornbread, pumpernickel, rye, and black bread. Bread has sometimes gotten a bad rap from health food aficionados, but this is appropriate only for that soft pasty confection known as American white bread. Real bread is a wholesome treat. Many men have found great satisfaction in learning how to make it.

It is well-established that people whose diets rely heavily on grains have fewer nutrition-related illnesses. Meals which are centered around a grain, such as rice, using meat only as a flavoring, are common in most of the world. The closer we come to following this diet, the better our nutrition. The shape and structure of human teeth suggests to scientists that we are designed as a species to be grain eaters, not meat-eating hunters. Have you seen any flesh-tearing fangs in the mirror lately? Instead, evolution has given us the grinding molars common to all other grain-eating animals.

VITAMINS

Although vitamin supplements have taken quite a beating elsewhere in this chapter, they sometimes do serve an important purpose. A well-balanced diet should provide us with all the vitamins and minerals we need, but there is little guarantee that our typical mass-produced foods contain all the nutrients that nature intends. Unfortunately, there is also very little hard information available on just what amount of vitamin intake is appropriate. The old government "minimum daily requirements" are widely criticized as out of date and unproven, but they are the only standards we have. Until something better comes along, they are useful guidelines.

Moderate use of vitamin and mineral supplements may be helpful and is not likely to be harmful. What's actually needed can probably be found in a single multivitamin or mineral tablet, though some would disagree. Taking 15 or 20 separate vitamin and mineral pills a day, though, is probably doing your local health food store more good than it is you. When vitamins are used, consistency is a good policy as it allows the body to adapt to what you're doing. Suddenly jumping from a little or no supplements to 10,000 mg. of vitamin C, for example, is more likely to produce diarrhea than healing. Some people suggest using *time-release* capsule of pills, 3,000 to 6000 mg. of vitamin C per day might be a reasonable supplement with little risk. Most vitamins are best absorbed when taken with food as they must combine with other molecules to be absorbed properly.

SPICES AND CONDIMENTS
The use of flavorings is particularly important when making changes in nutritional habits. It provides a great opportunity to experiment, even to have a little fun, while developing our epicurean talents. Start by throwing out the salt and the butter—the old staples—and bringing in the olive oil and garlic. Garlic, long noted for its ability to ward off vampires, is claimed to have many health benefits. At the very least, it makes for tasty food and seductive kitchen odors.

Using oil of any kind adds calories, so we must ever be watchful. The value or harm from saturated fats, such as butter, and unsaturated fats, such as vegetable oils, is hotly debated. Some contend there is a big difference, in favor of unsaturated fats, whiles others insists it doesn't matter in the least.

The money saved from a single missed restaurant bill should be enough to stock a worthy spice rack. Try to bring an experienced friend, one who cooks well, along to shop for spices. With a variety of choices on hand and the courage to experiment, it's easy to come up with new flavors and dishes to help cut down on the foods you want to cut back on.

Above All, Have Fun

Healthful food needn't be bland or weird tasting. Eating is one of life's pleasures and a healthful diet doesn't detract from that one bit. In fact, it adds to the pleasure when we know that what we're eating is actually good for us. A few simple tips can help make eating the fun it should be without the worry or guilt of poor nutrition.

1. PLAN YOUR APPROACH AND YOUR MEALS.
   Start with a review of your current eating habits. When and why do you pig out, eating too much or the wrong things? Once you know what events sets this off, you can plan your diet around them. Keep the kitchen stocked with the right things for the right times, so there's little need or opportunity for wildly incorrect meals. Try to plan your dinner menus in advance, in a clear and

deliberate state of mind, rather than walking blindly into the supermarket in a bad mood or after smoking a joint.

2. HANDLE EATING OUT WITH GREAT CAUTION
    Eating out presents one of the greatest challenges to good nutrition. Fatty foods are tasty foods, and the restaurant industry knows it. Fancy restaurants are quick to dollop on the rich buttery sauces, while inexpensive ones tend to fry things in animal fats. The safest approach is to eat out as seldom as possible, unless you can find a restaurant which as is sensitive to nutrition as it is to making money. There are quite a few places that seem to know what's good for us, but even they must cater to the masses. You'll still have to know what to order. Stick to the simplest, most basic items on the menu—salads (dressing on the side), vegetable dishes, sandwiches, grilled meats and fish. The more "gourmet-like" a menu item sounds, the more likely it is prepackaged, possibly even frozen. Ask for what you want or how you want it prepared, even if it isn't exactly spelled out on the menu. Ethnic restaurants often provide simple dishes based on beans, rice or noodles. A vegetarian burrito, for example, can be a very healthful dish.

    Eating in and bringing lunches from home also saves big money.

3. GET HELP FROM YOUR FRIENDS
    Let people know of your efforts and preferences when trying to improve your eating habits. If friends coming for dinner ask if they can bring something, be specific: *"How about picking up a few of those mangoes I saw at the Chi Chi market?"* They'll be relieved when they learn how little it costs compared to the chocolate torte or Dove Bars they had in mind.

4. KEEP A CLEAR HEAD
    As in sex, drugs and alcohol lower inhibitions and your commitment to better nutrition. Do your planning with a clear head. If you want wine, try saving it until after the meal, lest it influence what and how much you eat during the meal. If you must take a toke or two, make sure the cupboard is devoid of munchies.

5. SET A PROPER COOKING ENVIRONMENT
    Look at your kitchen. Is it set up to prepare wholesome meals or to unwrap TV dinners? If the cooking environment—the kitchen—makes food preparation difficult, you'll lean toward convenience foods. In a proper kitchen, it takes less time to steam vegetables than it does to zap a TV dinner. A few simple utensils and relatively inexpensive cooking gear is all that's needed.

6. FINALLY, DO IT FOR THE RIGHT REASONS
    We should eat to nourish ourselves, not to compensate for stress, hide from loneliness, or submerge our anger. If eating gets cross-linked with our emotional states, nutrition will suffer. Deal with the emotional states or stress in the proper way, and give eating and nutrition its proper due.

Eating right doesn't take a lot of money or time, and we don't have to become master chefs to do it. It doesn't require religious adherence to strange diets, unpleasant foods, or the endless use of expensive supplements and pills. Our digestive systems are quite flexible and adaptable and there is plenty of room for personal preference. Perhaps the biggest challenge we face is cutting through the commercial hype which surrounds the subject. People in countries where vitamin pills, mineral tablets, and bottled amino acids and proteins don't exist seem to get along just fine without them. What's needed is an adequate and balanced supply of natural foods, the kinds which grow in the earth, not test tubes.

Like altering our sexual practices, making changes in our eating habits may be a bit clumsy at first. With a spirit of adventure and a willingness to learn new ways and flavors, it can be an enjoyable adventure which serves as a sound foundation for all our other efforts at improving our health.

Rage and Helplessness

Sorting Out Our Feelings

Staying Alive, the Ultimate Political Act
(Making Medical Decisions)

Fighting Back
(AIDS Activism)

CHAPTER

7

FIGHTING FOR OUR LIVES

Preceding chapters of this book discussed key lifestyle issues which have an impact on our risk of contracting AIDS and on progression of the disease. This final chapter explores the fundamental threat of AIDS. Three themes are of the utmost importance:

- coping with the rage, helplessness, and emotional turmoil so many of us feel over the epidemic;

- making medical decisions which may affect our lives;

- taking a stand as a member of a community under siege.

Until we find a way to deal with the fury and anguish inside, we are not well equipped to face the challenges before us. Likewise, until we know who and what to trust, we cannot help but feel uncertain and indecisive about the critical medical choices we must make. When both our psychological and physiological houses are in order, we can address—as members of a community—the enormous hazards we face in a sometimes hostile environment.

RAGE AND HELPLESSNESS

Perhaps not since the Holocaust of World War II has a single group suffered in such a relentlessly focused manner. History records no other plagues confined within such clear social boundaries. Although the epidemic shows signs of slowly crossing over into the general population, the majority of those infected in most cities continue to be members of our community. Despite the rapid advance of AIDS in other minority communities, it will be a long time before any other community experiences the devastation we have already suffered.

Many are inclined to see conspiracy in our plight. After all, there is little doubt that our community is no favorite of the conservative administration in power during the developing years of the plague. The technology for creating a virus through genetic engineering perhaps became available in this decade. And the AIDS virus *has* been remarkably selective. Some theorists have presented well-constructed (though not well-documented) chronologies tracing the virus from secret laboratories to the streets of New York and San Francisco.

Others see only a conspiracy of benign neglect and bureaucratic bungling which took advantage of a bad situation. It is difficult to look at the federal and scientific response to AIDS and not wonder what the problem is, why every small step forward has taken so long.

Some, perhaps a minority, see little wrong and point out that progress against all viral diseases has been agonizingly slow.

No matter how we view the world's response to our plight, there is plenty to be angry about, both politically and personally.

POLITICALLY:

- It took years at the outset of the epidemic before the seriousness of the situation was acknowledged and addressed by authorities.

- Research was delayed for more than a year while battle raged over the legal and financial rights that came with discovery of the virus.

- Every increase in funding has required a tiresome fight by our lobbyists. Yet even now, funding remains inadequate.

- Our suffering is exploited by religious and political fanatics interested in blaming us for the problem, in condemning the victims, rather than finding a solution.

- National health agencies, despite years of funding from Congress, have failed to swiftly test potential treatments.

- Political opportunism drives federal agencies to divert money to no-win solutions, such as mandatory testing, contrary to the recommendations of public health officials and scientists.

- There is a growing federal trend toward writing off the 2 million or more already infected in favor of protecting those at least risk.

- Political and religious conservatives call for quarantine despite lack of evidence that it will produce even the slightest benefit.

PERSONALLY:

- We've seen friends and lovers suffer and die by the thousands while Washington scratched its head in indecision.

- We sit powerless in the face of regulatory agencies which block access to potential treatments which might at least give us grounds for hope; when treatments are finally offered, they come at a price which leaves many bankrupt.

- We face the dismal prospect of knowing that most people being diagnosed today (and for the next several years) were infected long before we knew of the problem.

- Our rights to privacy, our sexual liberties, and our freedom of movement are under attack as never before.

- Careers are shattered; housing and insurability are threatened by unreasonable and disproven fears of casual contagion.

Any gay man who isn't disturbed either isn't listening or isn't feeling. Most of us burn inside with indignation, yet seem unable to find a worthy target to strike out at.

For some, the flip side of rage is helplessness, the sense that nothing we do will make any difference, that we are victims facing insurmountable odds. We come to this perspective not solely out of psychological despair, but from a reading of the facts.

- For some people, research has added a few months of life, but is still unable to preserve it; some say we have only learned to prolong the suffering.

- Most researchers contend that no known science offers the hope of completely ridding us of the virus, and that, at best, those infected might be given a way to live with it.

- As our community is weakened by the loss of our finest brothers, homophobic groups grow in strength.

- The harder we fight against bureaucratic inefficiency, the more we learn that things have always been this bad and that even the smallest changes require a great deal of energy and effort.

- Even though the rate of new infection is dropping, hundreds of thousands of our brothers are still carrying a viral time bomb likely to explode within the next decade.

It's not surprising that many conclude that politicians won't help, doctors can't, and our friends and community are powerless against the great "gay plague."

Fight, Flight, or Submission

It would be easy to get hung up in rage and helplessness. Likewise, it's important to understand that our feelings have a basis in reality—we aren't crazy to feel what we feel. The question is what to do about it. However appropriate the feelings might be, they can be harmful to us if we don't do something about them. Internally, they take the joy and excitement out of life, leaving us preoccupied with all that is wrong, all that is working against us. This preoccupation can deeply affect our relationships. Moreover, unexpressed rage and helplessness produce additional stress with potential for ill effects on our health.

Our instinctive reaction under threat is the *fight, flight, or submission* syndrome well documented in most forms of life. Our fundamental choices are clear:

FIGHT:
> We can stand our ground and fight back in our own defense. A fighting stance *compliments*, rather than *contradicts*, acceptance of our plight as a community or a personal diagnosis.

FLIGHT:
> We can flee into denial, the opposite of acceptance. We can avoid discussion and acknowledgment of the threat, or willfully hide our real feelings with rosy views and positive platitudes.

SUBMISSION:
> We can give up and wallow in hopelessness, dwelling only on the harsh realities which provoke such feelings. If we are ill, submission will contribute to our earliest possible demise.

Other chapters of this book took pains to avoid telling the reader what to do. On this subject, the authors have a clear opinion: as individuals and as members of a community under siege, we owe it to ourselves and each other to choose to FIGHT rather than flee or submit. Flight and submission, whatever their appeal, leave us poorly equipped to combat illness on a personal level and shortchange the community in its battle with the forces marshaled against us. We must meet three challenges to succeed in this battle:

* SORTING OUT OUR FEELINGS (coping with emotions)
  First, we must tend to our own feelings and attitudes. We must know what we're feeling and how to cope with it. If we don't have our heads screwed on, our effectiveness will be minimal.

* STAYING ALIVE (making medical decisions)
  Next, we must choose a path for coping with the medical realities—to test or not test, to treat or not treat, to take charge of our own healing. *Staying alive is the ultimate political act.*

* FIGHTING BACK (AIDS activism)
  Finally, we must choose a course of action for meeting the challenges we face together as a community. As members of this community, we cannot idly stand by and watch its destruction.

CHALLENGE #1—SORTING OUT OUR FEELINGS

COPING WITH OUR EMOTIONS

For many, the hardest part of facing AIDS is coping with our emotional reactions to it. Strong feelings are inevitable when we are confronted with bad news. Lack of an emotional response often suggests an unwillingness to deal with the problem. Most of us experience varying degrees of fear, anxiety, anger, and sadness. Learning to cope with these emotions is the first step we must take to *fight*, rather than flee or submit. Doing so will help prevent more severe anxiety or depression or their flipside, emotional numbness. Similarly, our attitudes have a large impact on our response to the threat of AIDS. By carefully examining our attitudes and how they affect our feelings and our actions, we can cope more effectively with the demands placed on us.

Coping means handling our feelings, however difficult, and getting on with life. It does not mean that our problems disappear, or that our feelings of sadness, loss, or rage just fade away. One sign that our coping style needs improvement is an inability to overcome feelings of hopelessness, demoralization, or abandonment. When effectively coping, we experience confidence, a sense of being in control. We know we can handle whatever comes up.

Fortunately, in periods of crisis we see the full range of emotions—not just negative ones. Along with sorrow, pain, and suffering, we also experience love, courage, and joy, which spring from seeing ourselves in a nobler way. Emotions—feelings—are central to our humanity. They provide the hue and shade of our experience, the thunderstorms as well as the sunsets. But they are only one form of internal experience and they are distinct from our attitudes and thoughts. All of these are distinct from our behavior. Making distinctions between thoughts, behavior, and feelings helps us understand and cope with complex situations. We live by such distinctions. For example, it's not uncommon to have homicidal thoughts—*"I'll kill that son-of-a-bitch"*—but we seldom act on them. We are responsible only for our behavior, what we actually do. A few useful definitions:

EMOTIONS (feelings)	Internal sensations or perceptions—such as joy, sorrow, fear, hate—in response to events, ideas, or people. They often seem to have a life of their own. (*"I feel devastated! I'll never give my heart to a man again."*)
THOUGHTS	Internal comments or statements we make to ourselves—ideas and judgments inside our consciousness that exist in the form of language (words). (*"I think this would be a marvelous day to meet my prince in shining Levis."*)
ATTITUDES	Beliefs or positions we take regarding an issue, person, or thing; attitudes are usually conscious and include both our feeling and thinking responses to something. (*"Listen to the voice of experience: never trust a man who shops before noon."*)
BEHAVIORS	external actions; things we *do*. (*"I saw him in the crowd at Bloomie's, a friendly face in a sea of strangers. I smiled, he nodded back."*)

While it's not necessary to label every inner experience, having a common understanding of these terms makes it easier to diagnose problems in our response to AIDS.

Men and Feelings

Men in western society, including gay men, spend a lifetime learning to suppress their feelings. Our culture has long implied that feelings—emotions—are fine for women, but a sign of weakness in men. As boys, we learn that it is unmanly to cry, that we should accept disappointments without complaint, and that only girls express tenderness and warmth. Emotions are so closely associated with femininity that men who express them freely are suspected of being (gasp!) homosexuals. We often support this stereotype, automatically assuming that any sensitive man must surely be one of us (especially if he's good looking, famous, or both).

As a group, men have a difficult time recognizing and valuing their feelings. In recent years, a new, more sensitive role for men has evolved out of the enlightenment and experimentation of the Age of Aquarius. Although this "new man" is well recognized in magazine articles and books, the problem remains. Changing our beliefs about feelings doesn't automatically change our experience of them. Even in our community, where it is more acceptable for men to show their feelings, many of us still are out of touch with our inner selves. Feelings of love, tenderness, and understanding are fragile and sorely tested by the losses we are experiencing.

Coping with our feelings requires that we develop familiarity with our emotional patterns. Feedback from others can help, and thus, the ability to communicate about our feelings is very important. We gain nothing—and lose a lot—if we suppress our feelings. Our feelings are our feelings; we must learn to recognize, accept, and value them. They are never wrong or inherently bad. Any voice—internal or external—which tells us how we should or should not feel is in error. How we *act* on our feelings—our behavior—is where good and bad, should and shouldn't, do matter. Until we learn to experience our feelings, we can never really be ourselves.

Emotions Associated with AIDS

Facing AIDS evokes a full range of emotions. When hurt, we experience pain and much of that pain is emotional. If we cope in ways which allow us to continue to experience our emotions, we remain fully alive. When the pain becomes overwhelming, however, our defenses may step in to give us the necessary escape. If, however, we overuse our defenses, we become zombie-like, emotionally numb. At the other extreme, we can overindulge our feelings, allowing them to dominate our thoughts and impinge on every action. The challenge we face is to find ways to recognize and accept our feelings as they really are—without escaping into our defenses to hide from the pain—and without letting them govern our every move.

No more than we should ignore severe physical pain, should we allow ourselves to suffer continual emotional pain without help. Nor should we allow ourselves to live in a fantasy world of artificial "good" feelings or "positive" attitudes if, in fact, that is not our inner experience. To know when and how to act on our emotions, it helps if we can first recognize the problem. Several emotions which are commonly related to AIDS are described below.

ANXIETY:
Rollo May, a well-known psychologist, defines anxiety as "*...a feeling of uncertainty and helplessness in the face of danger.*" Anxiety, like stress, is neither good nor bad. A moderate dose helps us pay attention to what's going on inside and around ourselves. In larger doses, it produces very unhealthy results. Uncertainties regarding treatment, contagion, and progression of the disease make AIDS a ready and appropriate source of anxiety. On another level, AIDS renews questions about who we are, how we conduct our lives, and what it means to be gay. How we respond intellectually and emotionally determines how much of an impact anxiety has on us.

Given time, thought, and support, anxiety should ease. If anxiety becomes a lasting condition which yields little ground to reasonable clarification or a helping hand, professional help may be required. In rare instances, anxiety may have a physical component—perhaps due to a chemical imbalance—which must be treated medically as well as psychologically.

ANGER:
Anger has long played an important role in gay life. We eventually become angry at the discrimination and hatred directed at us. Learning to respect ourselves seems to require releasing our anger at those who make it hard on us. For most people, anger is the most confusing emotion. Popular wisdom warns of the danger in suppressing our anger, but we have also seen the harm that comes from giving it free reign and allowing it to rule our lives.

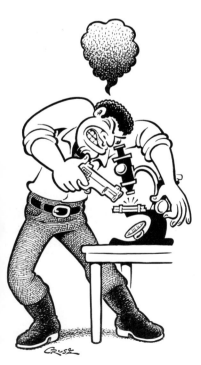

Now we face another threatening agent, a virus. As one man put it,

> "*How do you get angry at something that small? What can I do with the rage inside me?*"

When the object of anger is intangible, we turn it on ourselves or people we care about. A special danger for us is becoming angry at our gayness or the gay community. Both are ways of turning the anger on ourselves. Finding ways to express our anger is both helpful to us psychologically and crucial for the survival of our community.

GRIEF, LOSS, AND SADNESS:

Grief is intense mental suffering and distress, deep sorrow or painful regret, usually over the loss of a loved one. Legitimate grief is rampant in our community. Acknowledging and accepting our grief is an important part of mourning our losses and getting on with life. Ignoring or suppressing grief makes mourning more difficult.

Some losses brought about by AIDS are obvious and profound, others more subtle and harder to grasp. When we lose a friend or lover, we can't avoid the fact that a major event has occurred. Other losses, not so dramatic or clearly defined, still have an impact on us. For example, some people report a general sense of loss or sadness in the epidemic, even though they haven't lost friends or a lover. Their experience sounds a lot like grieving. They may be responding to a loss of sexual freedom or the sense of liberation we felt before AIDS.

Mourning the loss of a friend or lover, or even a cherished activity or freedom, takes time. Like a wound, it must heal. When loss is well defined and personal, grief can be intense and crippling. Sometimes, it begins before the death of the loved one and continues well after it. It may include periods of shock or emotional numbness, withdrawal, rage, weeping, and wide swings of mood and behavior. As time goes on, the swings become less severe, the peaks and valleys less intense. Grieving over the loss of a loved one often continues for as long as six months, even a year, before we are able to fully face life again.

When we experience a serious loss, failure to show the typical signs of grieving is usually a symptom of denial, a refusal or inability to accept the reality of what has happened. While grief stays bottled up and unaccepted, healing cannot be completed.

GUILT:

Guilt, a much maligned emotion, is a feeling that we have done something wrong. In a recent Gay Freedom Day parade, a sign read "GUILT IS THE ENEMY." Since most of us were taught that homosexuality is wrong, we grew up feeling guilty about our natural feelings of love and sexual attraction. Only by reevaluating our moral code were we able to overcome this double bind. In reaction to *inappropriate* guilt, some people decide that guilt is always wrong and try to eliminate the feeling completely. But guilt plays an important role. When working properly, it is a signal that we have violated our own ethical code. Like a gyroscope, it helps us stabilize and get back on our intended course.

Guilt presents a special dilemma for gay people: how do we know whether the guilt we feel is appropriate or simply a hangover from old teachings, social stigmas, and internalized homophobia? We can ask ourselves two questions to help determine whether guilt is appropriate or not:

Are the guilt feelings a response to breaking OUR OWN ethical code? (Are we feeling guilty because we broke our own agreement or is it a response to the voices of homophobia which still echo in our heads?)

Is the intensity of guilt we feel proportional to the violation?

The feeling of guilt is only appropriate when the answer to *both* questions is YES. It is entirely possible to do something which is wrong, even illegal, by society's rules, yet quite rightly not feel the slightest guilt about it. For example, being arrested for violating sodomy statues in Georgia may be an act of civil disobedience carried out with pride, not guilt (*"I did it solely as a matter of principle; didn't enjoy it one bit!"*).

Guilt can be a great teacher and a motivator. When we experience guilt and feel that it is appropriate, we must learn from it and *let it go.* If we get hung up on feelings of guilt, they torment us and the learning ceases. Learning to let go of guilt, even appropriate guilt, is one of the great lessons of maturity.

COURAGE AND HOPE:
Courage is not the lack of fear but the strength to face danger in spite of it. We see great examples of courage in the epidemic: people living with AIDS and ARC, people who stand by and care for them, people who fight against oppression and an unresponsive government. Another form of courage, often less noticed, is the courage to carry on with our lives in these troubled times, the courage to continue with everyday responsibilities despite the uncertainties we face.

Hope is the continuing expectation that something good will come out of our present situation. Even when hope of recovery from illness becomes unreasonable, this need not close the door to hope. We can still look to the future, to a time when this crisis will be over, perhaps to life on a higher spiritual plane, or to the love that will live on among our friends and families.

Hope can have real benefits in medical matters. It is so powerful that, when testing new drugs, science must take extreme measures to isolate its effects from that of the medication being tested. The healing power of placebos—inactive substances disguised as real medicine— is well documented. The value lies not in the placebo itself, but in the hope that it offers to patients and whatever healing powers of the body it unleashes.

People with hope, who retain a belief in their future, survive longest with AIDS. When hope is reasonable, we must share it freely with each other. Nothing is more demoralizing to a sick man than despair, whether from friends, family, lover, or doctor. We must sustain each other's hope rather than feed despair. When we give up hope, the body rapidly adjusts to our beliefs and the end comes quickly. The line between hope and denial, of course, can be a thin one. Research has shown, however, that both hope and denial give a person a better chance of survival than despair or hopelessness. Hope should not be lost until the patient himself makes that choice.

Just as loss and grief can stress the immune system, evidence suggests that courage and hope can enhance it.

If you wish, use the exercise on the next few pages to reflect on and describe the emotions you have experienced as a result of the AIDS crisis.

Emotional Diary

Instructions:

List your own *most significant* experiences of the *emotions associated with AIDS* discussed in the previous pages. For each you have felt, describe the situation which set off the emotion, its intensity and duration, and the effects it had on you.

ANXIETY

The situation: _____

_____

_____

Its intensity: *Mild*   *Severe*
                            1 ---------- 2 ---------- 3 ---------- 4 ----------- 5

Duration (how long you were affected by it): _____

Effects: _____

_____

ANGER

The situation: _____

_____

_____

Its intensity: *Mild*   *Severe*
                            1 ---------- 2 ---------- 3 ---------- 4 ----------- 5

Duration (how long you were affected by it): _____

Effects: _____

_____

GRIEF, LOSS, AND SADNESS

The situation: _____

_____

_____

Its intensity: *Mild*   *Severe*
1 ---------- 2 ---------- 3 ---------- 4 ---------- 5

Duration (how long you were affected by it): _____

Effects: _____

_____

GUILT

The situation: _____

_____

_____

Its intensity: *Mild*   *Severe*
1 ---------- 2 ---------- 3 ---------- 4 ---------- 5

Duration (how long you were affected by it): _____

Effects: _____

_____

COURAGE AND HOPE

The situation: _____

_____

Its intensity: *Mild*   *Severe*
1 ---------- 2 ---------- 3 ---------- 4 ---------- 5

Duration (how long you were affected by it): _____

Effects: _____

_____

Depression

Sometimes the pain of our emotions becomes so great that we shut down almost completely and suffer serious emotional disorders. The most common such disorder is depression. While depression might seem similar to the sadness everyone experiences from time to time, it can be a much more serious problem. If it lasts a long time or interferes with our ability to function in the "real world," professional help may be required.

What is depression? Mental health professionals use the term to describe a range of emotional states or conditions. These extend from a persistent sense of sadness or gloominess to extreme hopelessness, detachment, and despair. These feelings are often accompanied by:

- loss of initiative, loss of libido
- apathy or indifference
- insomnia
- loss of appetite
- thoughts of suicide

In extreme situations, frightening psychotic perceptions such as hallucinations may also occur. Since all of us facing AIDS experience some degree of dread, sadness, and rage, how do we know when this becomes depression? A few indicators:

- the length of time the feelings persist (*Is it just a bad day or two, or has it gone on without letup for a week or more?*)

- the persistence of self-hatred and feelings of guilt or worthlessness (*Are the feelings blatantly homophobic? Am I blaming myself, relentlessly, for the misfortune of others or my own past deeds?*)

- the degree of disconnection from everyone and everything (*Am I cutting myself off from the people in my life? Have I lost interest in the world around me? Am I spending my time alone, isolated, in silence—by choice?*)

If we face many of these feelings for long periods of time, we may be experiencing clinical depression. If so, a self-help book won't solve the problem. Talking things through with a counselor who is sensitive to the needs and concerns of gay people can often help in confronting depression and reducing the symptoms. When the problem is severe, medication may be needed to break the cycle of depression. At its most extreme, depression may require hospital care.

Suicide and AIDS
When someone contemplates suicide, he is asking the question,

"Does life have meaning any longer? Is it worth going on?"

In the face of death, this is a perfectly natural question. How we answer it may help us realize what is and isn't important in our lives.

Suicide has long cast a shadow over our community. Gay characters in literature and film, even when sympathetically portrayed, often come to tragic ends through suicide. Society has long used this tired image to frighten young people from expressing their gay feelings. As our community and our self-image have grown stronger, we have begun to correct this ugly myth. There is an excellent book on the subject of gay suicide: *I Thought People Like that Killed Themselves: Lesbians, Gay Men, and Suicide,* by Eric Rolfes (Grey Fox, 1983)

The media has exaggerated the problem with news stories that tell of persons with AIDS taking their lives in despair. Therapists who work with people concerned about AIDS note that, although many of their clients consider suicide, few take action. Even among those who experience severe pain, suicide is the exception rather than the rule. The occurrence of suicide among those infected with HIV is similar to those who are not: many consider it, few attempt it, and fewer still actually take their lives. Of those AIDS and ARC patients who have attempted or completed suicide, most suffered from severe depression. Others were influenced by drugs or alcohol.

There are, to be sure, some for whom suicide is a clearly chosen way of bringing their suffering to an end. Some who see an inevitable death in the near future choose not to live out their last days in agony, attached to life support machinery, or in a state of helplessness. Such a choice is quite different from that of someone who considers suicide out of depression. Some countries, in fact, legally permit AIDS patients to take their lives rather than demand that they suffer until the end.

Help is available in most cities through typical mental health services and suicide prevention hotlines. These services are usually staffed by nonjudgmental, caring people who can, if desired, refer a caller to a gay-sensitive therapist. Anyone considering suicide owes it to himself and his loved ones to consider this decision very carefully. If physical pain is the issue, the doctor can help bring it under better control. If emotional pain is the problem, therapy can help. Because there is no turning back, suicide must be thought through carefully in terms of its affects on loved ones. Survivors are often left with an undue burden of guilt—*"I should have done more."* Yet no one has the right to demand that a dying man endure unlimited pain or indignity to appease the feelings of loved ones or family. As in living life, ending it demands open communication to be fair to all involved.

Most people infected with HIV find meaning in their lives despite their illness. Some find renewed purpose in personal relationships and a growing sense of self-worth. Some find satisfaction in helping others and report that it provides relief from their own suffering. Anyone who knows or works with AIDS or ARC patients witnesses great dramas of love, compassion, and giving. For many, whether patient, soulmate, or volunteer, AIDS truly brings out the best that is in us. Living in the face of death has made our community more human, more caring, and wiser than it has ever been.

Internalized Homophobia

Homophobia, the irrational fear (and often hatred) of gay people, is deeply imbedded in our culture. Although some consider it a normal and moral state of mind, many psychologists now recognize homophobia, not homosexuality, as a mental disorder. When we as gay people show symptoms of this ugly disease, we call it "internalized homophobia." It is widespread in our community, although in a more subtle form than that demonstrated by obvious bigots. As children we were just as likely to be victims of anti-gay programming as anyone else. Internalized homophobia shows up in many ways:

• recurring guilt over our own behavior or sexual practices;

• unfair judgment about homosexuals who don't fit our own image—"butch" men who despise effeminate men, "disco queens" who can't stand "preppies" or 3-piece suits, gay men who stereotype lesbians, etc.;

• feelings of disgust or revulsion about the sexual practices of others—"tops" who look down on "bottoms" (except when they're in bed with one), "S&M" guys repulsed by "regular" guys, etc.;

• hiding "obviously" gay friends when the family's in town;

• gay activists and press who spend more time and energy attacking each other than the problems which confront our community;

• gay people who blame all their problems on the gay community.

Any time we find ourselves attacking other gay people, criticizing forms of expression within our community, or feeling bad about our own self-worth, it's time to ask whether we're suffering from internalized homophobia—and get off our own, or someone else's, case.

Religion and Homophobia

While some religious groups tend to the spiritual needs of gay people, others fan the flames of homophobia (and get rich while doing so). Homophobic hysteria has been a major fund-raising tool of many TV preachers (at least until they're caught with a mouthful of tubesteak).

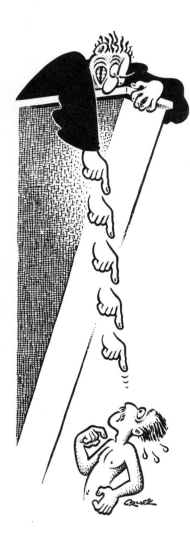

The fanatic ravings of religious bigots pick away at the kernel of homophobia which is present in most of us. Some of our brothers with AIDS have been deeply hurt by these vicious attacks and suffer renewed guilt over their previous lifestyle in their final, painful days. This appeal to internalized homophobia is a twisted distortion of religious belief. The Christian gospels report that Jesus saved his greatest condemnation for religious hypocrites, the "Scribes and Pharisees" of his day (the Falwells and Swaggarts of our day?).

The link between AIDS and our sexual practices rekindles old doubts and feelings of guilt we thought we had put behind after coming out. This has led some to renounce their gay identities and dwell in self-hatred. Instead, we need to better understand how internalized homophobia is an inevitable component of growing up gay, one that we can learn to overcome. *Gayness—homosexuality—is a naturally occurring and common form of human behavior.* It is present in all species, just as natural an occurrence as heterosexuality. Beyond that, all additional viewpoints are learned behaviors and beliefs, not natural or divine law.

Despite the raving of homophobic preachers, major religious books such as the Bible contain only minor and relatively obscure references on homosexuality. Where such references exist, they are hardly the main message and are typically found in the works of religious writers known for their extreme views on all aspects of sexuality (the letters of Paul in the New Testament, for example). The primary message of most religions is one of love and tolerance, not peer judgment and self-righteousness. Throughout history, the attitude of various religious groups regarding homosexuality has varied enormously, often reflecting the common practices of their day.

We cannot permit homophobia, internal or external, to add to our burdens in this time of crisis.

COPING WITH OUR FEELINGS

Learning to cope with our feelings, whether common emotions such as anger and joy, or the complex self-hatred of internalized homophobia, is a lifelong undertaking. Although there is no single formula for coping, there are several broad strategies which can be helpful.

Learning to cope—rather than hiding behind a happy face—pays off in several ways. First, the link between disease states and our emotional lives is well established. Effective coping results in less disease overall and less severity of existing diseases. The immune system is particularly responsive to emotional states. Secondly, the *quality* of life is improved when we are at peace with our emotions. Finally,

when we are healthier—physically and emotionally—we are better able to help in the battle against AIDS and oppression.

Perhaps the most important part of coping is just acknowledging what we feel. Any effort at recording, reflecting on, or discussing what we feel helps. We must avoid judging feelings—they are neither good nor bad, helpful or harmful. *They are just our feelings,* nothing more, nothing less. Although we are accountable for what we *do*— our actions, we cannot be faulted, nor should we fault ourselves, for feeling the way we do.

A second aspect of coping is realizing that emotions are transient, not permanent states. However bad we feel at any one moment, that feeling will eventually pass and give way to another. Knowing that a moment of pain, confusion, or anger will pass makes it easier to accept it. Even the deepest feelings, such as those experienced over the loss of a loved one, subside as our emotional wounds heal.

A third tactic of effective coping is learning to express our feelings. When feelings remain bottled up inside, we continue to be preoccupied with them. When we talk about our feelings with others— friends, lover, family, or counselors—the intensity of emotions often subsides. By talking things out, we better accept of our inner experiences and ourselves as we really are. Of course, sometimes talking alone isn't enough. Some people find relief in letting out a good scream now and then, or in pounding a pillow or punching bag, kicking a can, or relentlessly pumping on an exercise machine. As long we take care not to unfairly disturb others or hurt anyone (or ourselves), these more physical expressions are good ways to blow off steam and often leave us feeling better.

People who have lived for years with HIV infection often become experts at coping and have much to teach us. Despite illness, pain, and the limitations of an AIDS or ARC diagnosis, many live successfully and with fulfillment. Many such people learn to accept what is happening to them while finding a way to get on with life however they can. Their lives are infused with a shining clarity about what really matters and what doesn't, a purity of vision and values most of us seldom achieve.

A few observed characteristics of their coping style:

• They are "out" with their family and friends, both about their gay identities and their illness.

• They are able to acknowledge and express their feelings of love, fear, anger, and sorrow, without being overwhelmed by them.

• They make sure that life is worth living, allowing room for joy and stimulation, rather than dwelling on their illness.

• They achieve a balance of fighting spirit and calm acceptance of what is happening in their lives and live one day at a time.

Learning to cope is a lifelong challenge. A few general guidelines, such as those on the next page, can help when strong feelings become troublesome or cause us pain. While they are not a substitute for therapy, they can help us get through the ups and downs so common in this epidemic. The mere process of thinking things through, of acknowledging what we feel, makes a big difference in itself.

Guidelines for Coping with Emotions

1. **Identify and clarify the feelings.**
   Ask yourself, *"Just what am I feeling? Anger? Rage? Sorrow? Joy? How strong is the feeling? How long have I been feeling this way? Why?"*

2. **Allow yourself time to acknowledge and experience the feelings.**
   Accept the emotion without judgment, evaluation, or taking action. Just pay attention to what it feels like and how the feeling is affecting you.

   Most of the time, acknowledgment and acceptance of our emotional states, plus the passing of time, is all that's necessary. However, when emotions become so intense that they interfere with our ability to function, additional steps may need to be taken.

3. **Check the perceptions on which the feelings are based, preferably by talking things out with a friend.**
   Are the feelings proportional to the events on which they are based? Check your perceptions out with others. For example: If you're enraged about a roommate who *"always"* leaves a mess in the kitchen, check the facts yourself, or ask someone else. How often does he *really* leave a mess? If the answers seems disproportionate to your feelings, you might either *"get off it"* or find out what's really bothering you. Often, no one thing in particular is responsible for our emotions, but rather the combined weight of many things.

4. **Recognize feelings as a signal to pay attention to your internal and external world.**
   Ask yourself, *"What's happening, and do I need to do anything about it? If so, what?"*

5. **If action is required, do what must be done.**

6. **When you've done all that's reasonable, try to let go of the feeling.**
   Then try to relax. Accept the fact that you may feel bad for a while, but it won't be this way forever. Emotional states are transient and needn't be resisted, overcome, or suppressed. It is OK to feel bad, so let yourself do so—the feeling will pass more quickly if you do. The more we try to resist or fight our emotions, the more obsessed we become with them and the more they come to dominate us.

Coping with Uncertainty

One of the greatest agonies of AIDS is the uncertainty faced by the nearly 2 million people believed to be infected who have not yet fallen ill. People in support groups often report a sense of relief when a clear diagnosis is reached after years of vague symptoms and warning signs. Then, at least, a person knows what he's dealing with and what his options are. The long waiting period experienced by others can be a prolonged agony. As we've learned more about the epidemic and the increasing rate of progression to AIDS among those infected, the pain of waiting has grown.

For some, the waiting breeds hypochondria, in which every freckle is first seen as KS, each cough impending pneumocystis. Every morning begins with an apprehensive exam in the mirror, each month punctuated by a visit or call to the doctor. Some people literally worry themselves sick.

Many doctors now believe that HIV infection can be best understood and coped with as a chronic illness of varying but progressive intensity. People facing other chronic illnesses have learned a model of coping which can help us. Adapting this model to AIDS leads to a short list of productive guidelines:

1. GET EDUCATED: find the information you need.

2. CHANGE YOUR LIFESTYLE in the ways deemed necessary, such as those described in this book (sexual behavior, stress, etc.).

3. MONITOR YOUR IMMUNE STATUS, watching for signs that suggest a need for treatment.

4. ESTABLISH AND FOLLOW A TREATMENT REGIMEN as a routine part of your life.

5. GET ON WITH YOUR LIFE.

Coping with Mourning and Loss

One of the most widespread emotions associated with the AIDS crisis is the tremendous sense of grief and loss experienced. Many of us have lost close friends, lovers, and acquaintances. All share the loss of members of our community we may not have known. On a different level, most of us feel the loss of cherished activities and personal freedoms. When we are ill ourselves, we suffer losses in our careers, recreation, and our standard of living.

Few groups have ever faced the ongoing, repeated losses suffered now in our community. To find a comparable tragedy of on-going multiple losses, we must look to periods of wartime, the Holocaust, or the uncontrolled plagues of earlier centuries.

Whatever the depth of loss we feel, we must each find a way of adapting, a way to get on with our lives. J. William Worden, a psychologist, suggests that mourning involves four basic tasks we must accomplish to complete our periods of mourning.

1. ACCEPT THE REALITY OF THE LOSS.
    We must face the reality that a friend, lover, or community member is gone. In lifestyle losses, we must accept the fact that our health needs may require limitations on our sexual freedom.

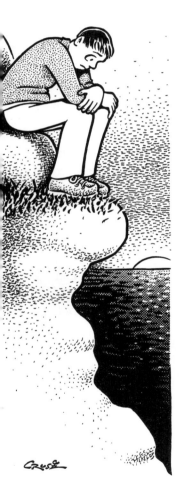

2. EXPERIENCE THE PAIN OF GRIEF.
    We must acknowledge the pain of loss. We can't hide from it or bury it in other activities. This doesn't mean, however, that we never get a break from the pain. There are times when it's inappropriate to dwell on our pain, times when diversion is a good survival strategy. What's required is a balance between acknowledging the feeling and paying attention to the other aspects of our lives. To achieve this balance, many have found it helpful to conduct rituals to memorialize a lost loved one. For example, some spend a few minutes each day remembering good times spent together or simply thinking about the loved one. By doing so, the pain of grief is given its proper time.

    Memorial services perform a similar function in the mourning process. They allow the friends and lover of the deceased to fully experience their loss and facilitate reinvolvement into every day life. Such ceremonies should commemorate the loved one in a personal and unique way, perhaps incorporating a specially favored activity or place. Elements which symbolize separation, such as the release of helium filled balloons which rise into the sky, are particularly helpful.

3. ADJUST TO AN ENVIRONMENT IN WHICH THE PERSON OR ACTIVITY IS MISSING.
    The difficulty in learning to adjust depends on the extent of our involvement with the person or activity. The loss of a lover may require a major restructuring of one's life. Likewise, if unsafe, anonymous sex was a common activity, we must give attention to finding safer ways to use our time.

4. WITHDRAW EMOTIONAL ENERGY AND REINVEST IT IN ANOTHER RELATIONSHIP OR ACTIVITY.
    The biggest difficulty here is in knowing when and how to do it. Some people try to move too fast and take a shortcut past tasks

1, 2, and 3. Others hold on, never wanting to let go of their past relationships or activities. Knowing when it's time to move on is always difficult. You know when you're ready when you're able to do it. Many of us need help to sort this out.

It's easy and understandable in a crisis such as this to shut down and become emotionally numb. The extent to which gay people have not withdrawn and continue to engage in life is a great testament to the courage, devotion, and spirit of our community.

Attitudes and Health

Attitudes are mental positions, beliefs, or viewpoints that we take toward other people, concepts, or events. They determine how we respond to events, how we judge them. In other words, our attitudes are how we look at things.

Attitudes are often associated with emotional reactions and tendencies to act in a certain way. Are we more likely to be open and accepting when we meet another gay person, a straight person, or a person of different color? Do we take responsibility for our health or do we prefer to allow others to make health decisions for us?

Attitudes are different from emotions. Emotions, such as anger, happiness, fear, and joy are more immediate and change more easily than attitudes. Attitudes build up over long periods of time in response to events and the feelings associated with them. We can change attitudes, of course, but doing so takes time and effort.

Some people try to suppress their true feelings in a misguided attempt to be "positive," or have a "positive" outlook. Strange as it may sound, there's nothing unusual about having a positive attitude along with negative feelings. An attitude is similar to the overall direction or course a ship takes. While the ship may encounter a storm and be thrown about, it can still stay on course. Similarly, we can maintain a positive attitude while experiencing emotional storms and still achieve our goals.

The extent to which attitudes affect our ability to fight off disease is widely debated. Similarly, the mechanisms by which they have an impact on health are unclear. The authors of the book *Getting Well Again* (Siminton, Bantam Books, 1978) suggest that attitudes play a significant role both in staying well and in recovering from all diseases. They point out that cancer patients, as a group, respond to problems and stress with a deep sense of hopelessness. They believe that this emotional response triggers physical processes which suppress the body's natural defenses and invite disease. Other health psychologists describe it differently. They believe that attitudes have an important impact on behavior, and that it is our behavior which in turn affects our health.

New research is now providing a better picture of the relationship between attitudes and how long a person survives when faced with a lifethreatening illness. In a study of patients with breast cancer conducted at King's College Hospital in London, the length of time patients survived after their diagnosis was shown to be related to their attitude toward the disease. Researchers grouped the patients according to four attitudes commonly expressed by people faced by threat of fatal illness:

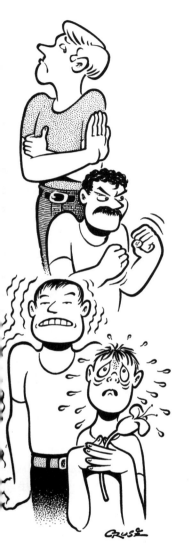

DENIAL -	*"I don't care what the doctors say. I never really had cancer."*
A FIGHTING SPIRIT -	*"I'm going to conquer this thing, fight it with all I've got!"*
STOIC ACCEPTANCE -	*"Keep a stiff upper lip, don't complain, be a man."*
HELPLESSNESS -	*"Nothing can be done. I'm as good as dead. There's no point fighting it."*

The study concluded that the group with the *fighting spirit* had the highest survival rate ten years after the diagnosis. Those who chose *stoic acceptance* or *helplessness* had the poorest outcome.

A positive attitude is the cornerstone of a sound health plan. Without it, our body's internal mechanisms can only work against us. A positive attitude can affect the course of disease or strengthen the immune system in several ways. It can:

• help *create the best possible environment* for fighting disease;

• *make the best* of a threatening situation;

• allow us to *focus all our resources* on supporting our health;

• *tap into little-understood powers* of healing within us.

While a positive attitude may help resist infection in these ways, powerful and destructive invaders such as the AIDS virus have strengths of their own. They may not bow easily to positive attitudes. If positive attitude alone were sufficient, there would be little need for the science of medicine. A sound health plan *must* incorporate the benefits both of positive attitudes and science.

The horror of AIDS makes it tempting for us to seek simple attitudinal solutions to the pain of illness, whether physical or emotional. Changing attitudes seems an appealing way to fix what ails us, since attitudes can indeed be changed. Yet it is this search for easy solutions which can lead us to over-rely on attitudinal healing and lead us astray. Unfortunately, the rapid devastation of AIDS makes quick solutions seem all the more attractive. After all, if they worked, who would want to take the time and trouble to do anything else?

Two popular *"quick-and-easy"* approaches which abuse the notion of attitudinal solutions:

SEE NO EVIL, HEAR NO EVIL, SPEAK NO EVIL
This one is as old as mankind. Regarding AIDS, it is a form of conscious denial. We don't want to talk about it, we tell our friends not to mention it in our presence, we are convinced it is only a problem "over there" in some other city or neighborhood, or among some other type of people. This view is often coupled with the fatalistic belief that nothing can be done anyway. When confronted with the reality that AIDS is all around us, this form of denial often gives way to hysteria and dangerously unbalanced behavior.

THE POSITIVE THINKING TRAP
We often try to reduce our feelings to simple notions of good and bad—love and happiness are good, anger and sadness are bad. Given a choice, we would prefer to stick to emotions like happiness and avoid unpleasantries like anger or grief. This can only be accomplished through suppression of our emotions. The underlying feelings don't really change, but we refuse to acknowledge the ones we don't like. Instead of being in touch with our inner selves, we become increasing detached and unrealistic. We come to wear the zombie-like smile of religious cult followers; we see only sunshine and flowers.

AIDS gives us all a lot to hide from, so it's hard to fault anyone for seeking refuge in positive thinking. But when forced positive thinking comes at the expense of honest self-awareness, we lose our ability to cope with even the simplest of problems. Life only works while the fantasy continues. When harsh reality comes our way—and the *"have a nice day"* fantasy crumbles—we are less able to cope than ever.

With good intentions, some AIDS support services have made a virtual cult of overvaluing positive feelings. It is true that we can do harm by dwelling on the negative, and there is proven value in looking to the bright side. Yet, it is equally harmful to paste on a happy face which simply doesn't deal with reality. Most who take this path do so only for a while and eventually return to a more balanced and realistic view of their situation.

Attitudinal healing can play an important role, especially in helping overcome deep-seated negative attitudes such as fatalism and hopelessness. We need reassurance that we are not mere victims of fate, that the outcome of our lives is a mix of fate, action, and will. Those who believe they can make a difference are able to do so. Likewise, attitudinal healing can help lift the burdens of guilt and doubt by restoring self-confidence and self-love. Attitudinal healing misleads us only when it is used as universal salve to smooth over the legitimate signals and messages our bodies and minds give us.

Getting Help

Most of us experience strong emotional reactions during times of extreme stress. While we can learn to cope effectively with a wide range of emotions, sometimes it is necessary to get help. There is no shame, no weakness, in seeking help, and a great deal of potential harm in trying to *"tough it out"* alone. Problems which might be solved easily working with a therapist can become more serious and gnaw at us for years if we fail to deal with them. In fact, there is great strength and maturity in knowing when to get help. To know when, we can ask a few simple questions:

1. *Are emotional reactions or attitudes interfering with everyday functioning at home, school, or on the job?*

2. *Are emotional reactions frequently excessive or disproportionate to what's happening? Is fear becoming panic, anger turning into rage, sadness giving way to depression? Are my attitudes seen as extreme or unreasonable by others?*

3. *Are emotions interfering with normal sleep patterns for an extended period of time (more than a week)?*

4. *Is there a consistent change in eating patterns? For example, is a loss of appetite leading to weight loss, or a surge in appetite leading to weight gain?*

5. *Do I have recurring thoughts of extreme actions, such as killing myself or others?*

6. *Are my attitudes and beliefs making it difficult for me to listen to others or accept the guidance of medical professionals?*

7. *Am I using drugs or alcohol to cope emotionally? For example, do I drink or use drugs to escape anxiety, depression, or fear?*

With each *yes* answer, the need for counseling becomes more evident. In selecting a therapist, it is important to choose someone who is sensitive to you as a gay person. While this often means a counselor who is gay, there are some therapists whose personal sexual preferences do not preclude their working sensitively with gay people. Good sources of recommendations include doctors, friends who have already seen counselors, AIDS community service bureaus, and local public health and mental health agencies.

There are dozens of widely held misconceptions used to avoid counseling—*"It's too expensive." "It takes years." "Psychiatrists are all crazy themselves."*—and so on. There's a good answer for every rationalization, and the bottom line is simple: it makes no sense to deny ourselves help when we need it.

Support Groups

Many people who don't feel a need for private counseling turn to support groups to help cope with the emotional demands of AIDS. Groups have been formed to serve all levels of need, including groups for people with AIDS or ARC, the "worried well," and friends, lovers and family of those who are ill.

Support groups provide an excellent opportunity to learn how others are coping with similar concerns and feelings. Just recognizing that others share such problems is a big help, as is seeing people at different stages of understanding and growth. Contrary to common misconceptions, being in a group doesn't mean spilling your guts to a bunch of strangers. The degree and kind of participation is up to the individual. Individuals take a variety of roles within groups. No one is under pressure to do anything they don't want to do.

As a special benefit, groups provide a great opportunity to meet new people with similar interests, concerns, and needs. For many people, support groups have taken over from the bars as a meeting place. Groups exist in almost every medium- and large-sized city. They can be located through the local AIDS service organization.

For all of us, getting our heads together is the first critical step in *fighting for our lives*. With a clear head, we can go on to make the necessary medical decisions to stay alive. And by staying alive, we can continue the fight for survival of our community.

CHALLENGE #2—STAYING ALIVE

MAKING MEDICAL DECISIONS

Despite concern over civil rights, lost friends, and diminished sexual freedoms, one issue overrides all others, yet it sometimes is not given the attention it deserves. The most fundamental threat we face is a medical one. If we fail to deal with it effectively, other concerns are meaningless. The need to make sound medical decisions, with a clear head, is critical to our survival as individuals and as a community. Unfortunately, the growing clamor we face over social and political threats sometimes clouds our vision, leading us either to overlook the medical issues or to view them from a distorted perspective.

Staying alive is the first and ultimate political act, the one most feared by our enemies. While nothing can make us completely free of the threat of AIDS once we've been infected, making the right medical choices will maximize our chances for survival, put us in the longest possible holding pattern while awaiting a cure, and ease the mental turmoil we face. To give it our best shot, we must learn to take charge of our medical situation. At the very least, this requires that we face the issues of testing and diagnosis, establish a strategy for choosing medical resources and treatment options, and grow in our ability to interpret medical information.

Choosing a Doctor

Before AIDS, few of us made a big deal out of choosing our physicians. If we were lucky, we found a gay physician we could be comfortable with. If we had serious problems, we were referred to a specialist—and that was that. In light of AIDS, we need to become very serious about whom we work with. A physician's experience treating HIV infection is a major factor in providing effective care. The availability of experienced doctors varies by location. It is no surprise that AIDS patients have a much longer life expectancy in some parts of the country than others.

The physician's attitude toward gay people also plays an important role in the quality of care and advice we receive. Physicians who are neither knowledgeable of nor sympathetic to gay lifestyles are less likely to provide the support we need. If their religious, political, or moral opinions find mere tolerance for us, or if they are ill with homophobia, we can expect routine care at best. In some cases, we get even less. When a doctor's beliefs include unreasonable fears of infection, care can become remote and detached. The patient knows it and withdraws into his illness.

Physicians who have primarily non-gay practices seldom accumulate experience treating the disease. Even though they may try to keep up with the medical journals, their capability is limited without practical, hands-on experience. All the technical information in the world can't make up for personal experience in the subtle ways of illness and healing. At best, the traditional sources of medical knowledge—journal articles and medical conferences—typically trail a year or more behind in reporting on the most advanced practices. New techniques and treatment options take a long time to work their way through the system.

Problems can exist even among physicians who are sympathetic. Doctors who have seen many men die of the disease sometimes develop their own fatalism and are no longer able to encourage their patients to keep fighting. Some of the busiest doctors have suffered severe emotional burnout from the epidemic. Their own sense of growing hopelessness is too easily recognized by their patients.

The best of physicians are aggressively interested in the progress of the epidemic and spend a great deal of their time learning and keeping up with the latest developments. They maintain personal contact with other physicians and researchers at the medical centers specializing in AIDS treatment. They learn from their own patients and community groups, who become understandably engrossed in following medical progress against the disease.

Friends, other physicians, and community support groups throughout the nation are good sources of referrals to physicians. Once we have a clear picture of what we need and want from a physician, it's increasingly easy to find one.

The Healing Partnership

AIDS, like other critical illnesses such as cancers, causes us to examine the responsibilities of ourselves and our doctors in the healing process. Patients of Western medicine have often fallen into a very passive role, expecting the doctor and whatever pills, surgery, or high-tech magic he or she uses to handle the healing process. The patient's role is often simply that of bill payer. This works fine until we encounter a disease that doesn't respond quite so willingly to this model.

In *Anatomy of an Illness* (Bantam Books, 1979), Norman Cousins tells of his successful fight against a usually fatal disease. With the help of his doctor, he took an active, positive approach to his health. When later asked what conclusions he had drawn from the experience, he replied:

The first is the will to live is not a theoretical abstraction, but a physiological reality with therapeutic characteristics. The second is that I was incredibly fortunate to have as my doctor a man who knew that his biggest job was to encourage to the fullest the patient's will to live and to mobilize all the natural resources of body and mind to combat disease. Dr. Hitzig was willing to set aside the large and often hazardous armamentarium of powerful drugs available to the modern physician when he became convinced that his patient might have something better to offer. He was also wise enough to know that the art of healing is still a frontier profession. Although I can't be sure of this point, I have a hunch he believed that my own total involvement was a major factor in my recovery.

Most medical professionals readily admit that, for the most part, the body heals itself. Science, medicine, and doctors simply assist in the process. Physicians give us confidence, assurance, and belief in our ability to heal ourselves. Some preachers claim to heal in similar ways. As we face more deadly or complex diseases, we come to expect more science and less psychology or magic.

People who face life-threatening illnesses sooner or later come to realize that the doctor's power is limited. With AIDS, it is very limited. Thus, we face the question of whose responsibility it is to heal us. A list of the "powers" which combine to produce healing might realistically include (not in order of importance):

- THE TECHNOLOGIES OF MEDICINE: drugs, vaccines, surgery, diagnostic machinery, and life-support systems which act to permit the body to heal itself despite invading organisms.

- THE WILL, ATTITUDE, BEHAVIOR, AND KNOWLEDGE OF THE PATIENT: positive attitude, the will to live, health-conscious behavior, and knowledge of the patient all promote healing. Fatalism, passivity, ignorance, and self-destructive behavior don't.

- THE ATTITUDE, KNOWLEDGE, AND TECHNIQUES OF THE PHYSICIAN (and medical support personnel, such as nurses, therapists, counselors, etc.): a positive outlook which supports the possibility of healing is essential; the physician's knowledge (sometimes augmented by the patient's) is necessary to effectively coordinate the other tools of healing. Going beyond clinical techniques and offering one's humanness, including touch, seem to have an unexplained but powerful role in the healing process.

Healing occurs when these powers work in harmony. If the patient takes a completely passive role and assumes his doctor will cure him of AIDS, he will be sadly disappointed. A coordinated partnership is the most effective working relationship in situations such as AIDS, where no one source of healing has all the power. As patients, we must be willing to work with the doctor, not against him or her. The doctor must be willing to engage in partnership with us. Ultimately, the patient is in charge, since it is his life which is at stake. Most doctors are sensitive to this need and agree to work with the patient in whatever way is desired. The specific roles are subject to negotiation, based on the capabilities and styles of patient and doctor.

In a healing partnership, as patients we must:

• Follow the doctor's orders once an approach is agreed upon.

• Report openly and thoroughly on sensations, symptoms, signs, and feelings.

• Understand and accept the doctor's limitations, without blaming him or her for the outcome of shared decisions.

• Be clear about expectations, desires, and preferences.

It is critical to remember that the doctor is human too, with feelings and needs like the rest of us. A smile, an acknowledgment for the care he or she has given, and a willingness to forgive human failings, will go a long way toward enhancing the care we receive.

As patients we have a right to expect the doctor to:

• Explain the WHAT and WHY behind important options, permitting the patient the opportunity for fully informed consent.

• Invite or encourage second opinions, without repercussion.

• Respect the patient's knowledge and right to ultimate control.

• Share in the patient's hope and vision of a future until one is no longer possible.

• Estimate each patient's chances individually, without demoralizing us by the use of statistical norms.

Many times we can improve the quality of our care by showing greater consideration for the complexities of a doctor's schedule. For example, many people wish to know the what and why behind every recommendation the doctor makes—a practice which can conflict with a doctor's need to see everyone else on his or her schedule. We can minimize the potential for disruption, and increase the chances of getting what we want, by planning each visit in advance, listing ahead of time the key things we want to know and discuss. This can be communicated to the doctor in advance of an appointment, thus making it possible to schedule as much time as will be needed.

When we feel we're not getting the kind of care we need from the doctor, the first step to correct it is to let him or her know what's wrong. We can't ask doctors to read our minds, and it's unfair to expect them to correct problems in the relationship without knowing what they are. If, in the end, it becomes clear that the doctor can't or won't give the kind of care preferred, most physicians will assist us in changing doctors with dignity and no hard feelings.

AIDS Antibody Testing

Few subjects raise as many complex emotions and disagreements as that of antibody testing—the "AIDS test," as it is incorrectly called. The degree of conflict makes it difficult to make a responsible decision or even see all the arguments clearly. In virtually any other disease, diagnostic testing is simply a medical issue. AIDS antibody testing, however, is also a political issue and a psychological issue. To make a choice we can live with, we must face the test on each level.

THE POLITICAL ISSUE:
Rightwing political and religious leaders have placed mandatory testing and quarantine at the top of their agenda for combating AIDS. Their motives are transparent and hardly new: push back the hard-won civil liberties of gay men and lesbians. This approach has been opposed by nearly every public health leader and AIDS expert in the country. Yet the momentum for forced testing grows ever louder. Many gay people have come to fear that the record of a positive antibody test might someday—soon—be used against us. If we don't trust the political motives or intentions of government, we don't want our test results in their hands.

THE PSYCHOLOGICAL ISSUE:
The decision to test or not test carries certain psychological risks, ranging from mild emotional distress to hysteria and depression. There are even reports of suicides among people who learned of positive test results without adequate counseling.

In the early years of the epidemic, some health professionals believed that few who were infected would develop AIDS and argued that since no treatments were proven helpful, little could be done about a positive test result. Thus, they concluded that "ignorance was bliss," that the risks of testing (anxiety, depression, possible suicide) outweighed the benefits. Some recommended testing only for people who needed additional incentive to change sexual practices. In contrast, others pointed out that knowing your antibody status helped motivate lifestyle changes, helped guide decisions about the future. They argued on behalf of the greatly lowered anxiety which followed a negative test result and the potential benefits of promising but not unproven treatments.

Accumulating evidence shines new light on these issues. Long-term studies now suggest that the majority of those infected will eventually develop symptoms of ARC or AIDS. Also, helpful treatments which meet government approval are now available and there is a rapidly increasing emphasis on treatment at the earliest signs of disease. These factors are causing reappraisal of the risks and benefits of testing by those who have chosen against it in the past.

THE MEDICAL ISSUE:

There is little debate when testing is viewed solely from a medical perspective; like any other illness, early diagnosis of HIV infection is very important. It alerts people to the risk of transmitting disease, the increased danger from picking up co-factor illnesses from others, the need for health-promoting lifestyle changes, and the need to seek early treatment intervention.

To the old adage that *"Nothing can be done about the infection anyway, so why get people upset?"* many insist that much can be done and that this has always been the case. There is little argument that the fight against HIV can be enhanced by lifestyle changes, such as stress reduction, exercise and nutrition programs, safe sex, improved social support, and counseling. Once a person knows he's infected, he may need to take an even harder look at lifestyle issues (*"Should I add stress by taking that new job? Is it time to really cut down on drinking? Should I work fewer hours, take more vacations?"*)

Approved treatments were at first available only to those who were most ill. While awaiting a real cure, thousands of people have pursued promising, if not fully proven, treatments long before they faced serious stages of the illness, usually with the support of their doctors. *"Why wait until I'm dying to begin treatment?"* they ask. Indeed, there are no other diseases for which treatment is withheld until the patient is nearly dying. Once promising medicines make it through the lengthy government approval process, treatment at the earliest stages of HIV infection will almost certainly become a reality. Antibody testing is the first step in that process.

In the early years of the epidemic, *"Wait and see"* was often the advice of physicians faced with the uncertainties of AIDS. Today, we know very well what happens when we *"wait and see."* The minute serious symptoms are evident, nearly everyone gets tested anyway, so, some argue, what's the point of waiting?

A Personal Solution

Although there is a growing tide of opinion in favor of *anonymous voluntary* testing, we must each make our own decision. We must consider *all three* major issues—political, psychological, and medical. Making a choice that overlooks the medical value of testing is an unnecessary gamble with our lives; ignoring psychological factors risks our sanity; disregarding the political threat may save our health at the expense of our freedom. A few points which are essential for anyone considering testing:

PRIVACY:
Confidentiality must be *assured.* Promises by officials or even a trusted doctor may not be good enough. Politics have a way of overruling good intentions. The safest approach is anonymous testing. This is available on request in some states, and the mechanism guarantees anonymity. People who submit blood samples are identified only by a code number *of their own choosing.* The testing authority *never* has the name, address, or phone number of the person being tested. In states where anonymous testing isn't offered, gay people have found other solutions. Proof of identity is not normally required, so it is quite easy to use a false identity. Sympathetic physicians often cooperate in such efforts, but even at worst, an unknowing and unsympathetic physician can be duped into assisting.

An actual diagnosis of AIDS almost always compromises privacy since it must be reported to public health agencies in many states, and it is at least noted in medical records. To date, there are very few reports of hospitals or physicians making inappropriate use of this information.

COUNSELING:
No one should take the test without counseling, period. Many states provide this automatically. Gay service agencies in nearly every major city provide referrals to gay-sensitive counseling. New methods of "testing by mail" may prove dangerous if they result in people getting test results without counseling.

Most people who take the test learn to cope with the results. For many, the test proves negative and provides enormous relief. A NEGATIVE TEST RESULT, THOUGH, SHOULD ALWAYS BE CONFIRMED BY A SECOND TEST. To guard against *"false positives,"* positive tests are routinely checked and rechecked without the person ever knowing it.

The most effective approach to counseling includes discussions both *before and after* testing. A few important points which ought to be discussed in every counseling session:

• Before testing, learn just what the test does and doesn't mean (a positive result means a person has come in contact with the virus and should consider himself capable of passing it on to others; it does not mean the person has AIDS or will necessarily come down with AIDS).

• How will you cope with the emotions produced by the test? Who will provide support?

• What implications will the test have in your relationships? Discuss it *beforehand.*

• What steps should be taken as a result of the test result—medical and lifestyle?

INFORMATION

Once a positive test is confirmed, we can tune into the vast resources created by and for gay people facing this epidemic. There are resources for counseling, support groups, physician referrals, information on approved and unapproved treatment options, access to clinical drug trials, legal and financial support and counseling—to name just a few.

The following page summarizes the arguments for and against testing. Use it to make your own decision taking all factors into account.

Arguments Against Testing

Loss of privacy: test results might be used against us by insurance companies, employers, or bigots seeking quarantine.

Adverse emotional impact, including suicide: knowing might cause severe emotional stress (for the individual or within a relationship), which will make the disease worse. Knowing will drive a person crazy.

The test is inaccurate and its meaning unclear; it doesn't tell whether a person has AIDS or will get it in the future—so why bother? It will only lead to more anxiety and confusion.

There is nothing a person can do about a positive test result anyway, so why bother? Most people are already engaging in safe sex. Most have already made all the lifestyle changes they can.

"My doctor says nothing helps."

"I know I'm positive—I must be. The test won't make any difference."

Although some treatments exist now, better ones will be available later. Why take a chance with what's available now? Ineffective treatments might make things worse. It might be better to wait for the newer ones.

Counter-Arguments in Favor of Testing

Anonymous testing is almost always possible using "anonymous test sites" or phony names.

Counseling is essential—don't take the test without it. The stress of knowing can be overcome; damage done by the unchecked disease process cannot. HIV infection is an unpleasant reality that is better faced than denied, however painful that may be.

The test has become very accurate but should always be confirmed by a second test. If positive, it means the person has come in contact with the virus, should be considered contagious, and has a high chance of developing some form of the disease over the next 10 years. When symptoms are present, it helps doctors confirm the diagnosis.

The test helps overcome indecision and get on with self-preservation. Most people claim they are motivated to make additional changes: lifestyle changes to prevent contagion and to protect oneself from other diseases; testing of the immune system to estimate the stage and progression of disease; evaluation of risks and benefits of early treatment.

Get a new doctor.

Many discover otherwise. Testing, not intuition, is the only way to know.

No one knows when better treatment will be available; we have been repeatedly disappointed in this regard. Precious time may be lost, allowing the disease to reach a more serious stage when treatment is less effective. There is enough information to avoid harmful treatments. To date, no widely accessible treatment has been as harmful as AIDS itself.

Coping with Medical Test Data

As more and more people have tested positive for HIV infection, great interest has developed in medical tests which measure the strength of our immune systems. Intended originally for use by physicians, such tests have now become common dinner table conversation. Properly used and understood, they are useful and important. Misunderstood or overapplied, they can do a great deal of harm. This type of testing presents a dilemma for doctors and patients alike:

- While doctors need data to monitor patients' progress, the clinical and predictive significance of many tests is uncertain.

- Abnormal values on test scores don't always correlate to what the patient feels physically; telling the patient can sometimes set off harmful psychological reactions.

- Test results vary widely from one lab to the next; *unless the same lab always does the testing and consistent procedures are followed,* there is little comparability in the results, and thus only minimal value in the testing.

- Some tests are imprecise and the values unstable even in healthy patients; people experience unnecessary mood swings when they evaluate their condition solely by such measures.

- Patients don't always have the knowledge to know what is normal, acceptable, or ominous in test data; it's easy to become overly alarmed or inappropriately unconcerned.

Some doctors prefer not to do any more testing than is absolutely necessary and to carefully screen the information which is given to patients. This may be fine with some patients and infuriating to others, especially those who seek a strong role in their own healing. Other doctors have more regard for testing and educate their patients about what the numbers mean. This may be very satisfying to the more active patients, but confusing to those who prefer to leave things up to the doctor.

Whatever the doctor's personal style, people have a right to expect cooperation with their wishes. If that means frequent testing and openness about data, even if the doctor prefers otherwise, we have a right to demand it. For those who are more willing to trust their feelings about what is going on in their bodies, the doctor can be expected to monitor things prudently and interrupt the patient's perceptions only when the data demands it.

Some of the questions we face over this type of testing are similar to those of antibody testing:

- *How will the test results be used?*

- *Does knowing make things better or worse?*

- *What does the test mean, and not mean?*

- *What, if anything, should be done about the results?*

In every instance, both patient and doctor must be clear on these points, and many critical test results should only be released along with counseling. Without counseling, it's all too easy for us to experience unnecessary anxiety and start letting the tests, instead of our bodies, tell us how we feel. The more experienced we become and the more we learn from our doctors and other resources about the tests, the greater our chances of having a balanced view of medical diagnostic tools.

T-cell Testing

One test which is widely used to measure the health of the immune system is the T-4 cell count. The test measures the number or count of a certain type of white blood cells, T-4 or *helper* cells, found in a fixed amount of our blood. This number is important because the T4 cells are a primary target of the HIV virus. The virus invades these cells, takes them over and uses them to produce additional virus, and eventually kills the original cell. This is critical since the T-4 cell is one of the primary mechanisms of the immune system, one of the cells which normally helps us fight against an infection such as HIV. The HIV virus's ability to infect these cells is one of the reasons AIDS is such a difficult and deadly problem. As HIV infection progresses towards the AIDS condition, the number of healthy T-4 cells typically falls. Falling or abnormally low T-4 cell counts are a strong indication that the immune system is breaking down.

A completely normal count is 800 or more, a count above 500 or 600 is usually considered to be in the "safe" zone, and a count consistently below 200 is commonly associated with AIDS or near-AIDS condition. Many doctors use this test on a quarterly or semiannual basis to monitor the health of ARC patients or people who are infected but not showing any symptoms of disease.

While this might suggest that everyone should run out and get a T-4 cell count, science has learned that there are important limitations to this test. Most doctors treating HIV infection have one or more patients with full-blown AIDS despite high T-4 counts and others with low counts who resist development of AIDS or experience only mild symptoms. At best, the accuracy of this test is thought to be plus or minus 100 points and the results vary widely from one lab to the next. A high count one month at one lab may be followed by a low count next month at a different lab—when in fact the patient's condition hasn't changed at all. During periods of infection and for other reasons not well understood, the T-4 cell count seems to vary widely.

It's all too easy, and often damaging, to use this one test result to measure our overall condition. A more reasonable strategy for using and interpreting T-4 cell counts might include the following points:

IN GENERAL:

• Make sure that T-cell testing is always done by the same lab; going to the same doctor doesn't necessarily guarantee this unless it's specifically requested.

• When a low count is found, repeat the test immediately to rule out a fluke in the testing process; such flukes are very common. REMEMBER, it is the *overall trend*, rather than the count on any single test, which is relevant. A single surprisingly low test number means little by itself; when this occurs, the test should be repeated. Keeping a personal chart or graph of the numbers over time is helpful.

• In judging the significance of the test results, be sure to consider any other factors which might influence the test, such as periods of extreme stress or other infections.

SERO-POSITIVES (HIV positive but without symptoms of illness):

• Quarterly or semiannual T-cell testing can be a useful indicator of changes or decline in the immune system. When the number appears to be falling, or consistently stays below 500, treatment options, approved and unapproved, might be discussed with a physician. Community resources and many physicians can provide information on what the options are, including anti-viral therapy (to stop the spread of the virus) and immune boosting therapy (to strengthen the immune system).

ARC (people with symptoms of HIV infection):

• Quarterly or semiannual T-cell testing can monitor changes or overall decline in the immune system. If the number stays below 500, reaches as low as 200, or simply doesn't go up much anymore, treatment options definitely should be discussed with a physician. Some "approved" anti-viral treatments become available to people when the T-4 cell count reaches a certain lower threshold, such as 200. Some such treatments appear to produce lasting, but relatively small improvements in T-4 cell counts for ARC patients.

People whose counts consistently fall below 200 might consider *preventive* treatments against the possibility of particular opportunistic infections, such as pneumocystis pneumonia.

FOR PEOPLE DIAGNOSED WITH AIDS:

- Monitoring of T-cell activity becomes less important, since all medical precautions are likely to have been taken already. The results of the test are unlikely to lead to any changes in therapy. Patients must weigh the psychological risks of monitoring their health "by the numbers" against any possible benefit of T-cell testing. For people who successfully live with AIDS for long periods, annual T-cell testing may be prudent.

    T-cell testing may be a helpful measure of the effectiveness of treatments or experimental therapies, but as of 1987, no approved treatment has shown a consistent ability to produce lasting T-4 cell improvements for AIDS patients.

In all of these situations, it is important to understand that the test values are only approximate, not rigid, infallible indicators. The physician's interpretation is important since it takes many other factors into consideration. Similarly, a physician who has seen the random rise and fall of T-4 cell counts in many patients can help ease undue concern over changes in this number.

On the bottom line, most physicians and researchers consider this test to be an important measure of the health of our immune systems, but not the only one. Its value lies in giving clues about the best time to start treatment and what treatment strategies to use. Monitoring this or other test results only becomes a problem when the numbers simply add to a patient's anxiety.

The most serious abuse of this test occurs when insurance companies, prohibited by law in many states from using the AIDS antibody test to screen applicants, use the T-cell test as a substitute. Although "normal" applicants are never required to take the test, people who fit a certain profile—single males between the ages of 25 and 50 who live in urban centers—are increasingly forced to take the test as a condition of insurability. This is extremely unfair because of the inaccuracies of the test and the many variables other than HIV infection which can produce a low count.

Treatment Strategies

As yet no treatment is a cure for AIDS or ARC. There is strong evidence, however, that available treatments can slow the progress of the disease, help combat opportunistic infections, and, to some extent, strengthen the immune system. There are at least three distinct problems which must be addressed by a treatment strategy. First, something must be done about the spread of the virus in the body. Secondly, the body must be protected from infections which attack because of a weakened immune system. Finally, something must be done to restore the immune system. Some researchers also believe there is an "auto-immune" aspect to AIDS as well, a problem in which a diseased immune system begins to attack the body itself.

ANTI-VIRAL THERAPY:

If unchecked, the virus continues to take over new cells and produce additional virus. Eventually, all the helper cells of the immune system are crippled or are being used to produce new virus. Anti-viral drugs do not kill the virus itself, but instead interfere with the virus's ability to reproduce. Different anti-viral drugs interfere at different stages in the virus's reproductive cycle, but all share the goal of stopping the spread of the virus to new cells and the production of new virus. Even if a drug were 100% effective at this (none are), some virus would remain in cells already infected. In addition, it is believed that the virus infects cells in the nervous system and brain, so an effective anti-viral drug must be able to cross over into the brain and spinal fluid. This is a very difficult task for most drugs, since the brain is normally well-protected from substances in the blood.

Today's anti-viral therapies typically interfere with the body's most basic processes of cell reproduction and are thus capable of producing undesirable side effects. The most effective ones will be those which best slow reproduction of the virus while producing the least severe side effects. Side effects from the one currently approved drug ranges from nonexistent for many people to severe for others. In some cases, the side effects can be worse than the disease. On balance, though, anti-viral therapy has been proven to help many AIDS patients and this holds open the promise of more effective drugs in the future. Anti-viral drugs should be able to slow the progress of the infection in ARC patients, preventing or at least delaying the onset of AIDS. This effect, already demonstrated in preliminary research, offers exciting hope for people in early stages of the disease.

IMMUNE-BOOSTING THERAPY:

Anti-viral therapy on its own has not been able to restore the immune system of people with AIDS. Some small improvement has been shown in ARC patients, but researchers disagree as to whether the improvement is significant. Another class of drugs, called *immune boosters* or *immuno-modulators*, is under study which seem to act directly on the immune system. These drugs may be able to help the body itself combat the virus more effectively. Most researchers believe that these drugs should be used in combination with anti-viral drugs, thus slowing the virus while rebuilding the immune system at the same time. Although this belief has been common for years, research is only now beginning to test such combinations.

TREATMENTS FOR OPPORTUNISTIC INFECTIONS:
Most people who die from AIDS are not killed by the virus, but by other infections. Most, such as the one which causes pneumocystis pneumonia, are caused by common organisms which the body normally has little trouble fighting off. When the immune system is damaged, the body loses the ability to fight back. Various treatments are available for these infections, but they require some degree of help from the body's natural defenses. Eventually, when the body has no resistance left, even the best treatments are ineffective.

Sources of Treatment

There are three ways to obtain anti-viral and immune-boosting drugs. One is to try government-approved drugs, such as the anti-viral drug AZT, which has been shown to slow spread of the virus and extend life. Although this may sound like a perfect solution, the drug is not yet available to people at all stages of infection, is very expensive, and produces unacceptable side effects for many people. As of 1987, only one anti-viral—AZT—and no immune-boosting drugs have been licensed for use against HIV infection.

A second way is to seek access to drugs which are still being tested prior to government approval. These drugs may offer the hope of fewer side effects or greater effectiveness. Access to them is generally available only by volunteering as a subject in a clinical research trial. This approach also offers free medical care during the trial and for some time afterward. There are no guarantees, however, and some people have been seriously hurt in such experiments. However, now that better treatments are becoming available, the likelihood of receiving a very harmful drug is greatly diminished. After an agonizingly slow start, large numbers of openings in such trials are finally becoming available. Before volunteering, it is always best to weigh the overall risks and benefits of a particular trial with a physician who knows one's medical history and prognosis.

Volunteers in clinical trials provide critical service to the rest of the community. We would have no approved treatments today if not for their courage and personal sacrifice. Those who died or suffered as a result of early trials are heroes in the war against AIDS.

Thousands of AIDS and ARC patients and people who are sero-positive have felt enormous frustration with the slow pace of government approval of drugs. This has led to the creation of a virtual AIDS underground across the nation which supplies information about (and sometimes, access to) unapproved but promising treatments. Some are drugs under study in clinical trials, some are "generic" equivalents of experimental treatments or "non-drug" medicines bought from a variety of sources, and some are experimental drugs which are available in other countries but not in the U.S. Although not all doctors approve of the use of such treatments, most consent to monitor patients who use them, and some are active supporters of the AIDS underground. Resources which supply information on unapproved treatments are listed in the Resources Appendix of this book. Enormous expertise has developed in the gay community to meet the need for treatment in the absence of "official" solutions. Community wisdom accumulates based on reports of what is working for people and what isn't. Although such information is anecdotal rather than scientific, its validity is enhanced if the positive experience is repeated by large groups of people.

Most groups—both traditional and underground—believe that combined anti-viral and immune-boosting therapy is required. All treatments currently available are limited in capability and at best buy time or stabilize a patient's condition until better solutions become available. There is also a growing observation that no one treatment or combination works for everyone. To some extent, each person must work with his doctor to find and monitor the solution which seems best for the individual. Whenever approved treatments are available, they seem to be the logical place to start.

When underground treatments are tried, it's particularly important to know what you are buying and from whom you are buying it. Such treatments are often not produced under the same controls as licensed pharmaceutical products. Buying cooperatives and advisory groups have sprung up around various treatments to moderate the prices charged and monitor the quality of the product. When no such group is available, the buyer must beware on his own. Many of us have come to be quite cynical, perhaps with justification, about the slowness of the traditional medical establishment to offer help, and we have learned to ask tough questions of our doctors. We owe it to ourselves to be at least as cynical and demanding when experimenting with treatments from the local health food store or buying white powders and untested solutions from strangers with a profit motive. This doesn't mean that underground solutions should be ignored, since large numbers of people have found help there. But we need to be wise consumers, no matter from whom we buy.

A few questions to ask of anyone offering a hopeful treatment:

- *What evidence is there that the product works, and what is known about its side effects?* Insist on reading all available scientific literature, and asking your doctor to read it as well. If you don't understand it, get help.

- *What is being done to get the product licensed for use?* If nothing, there's probably a good reason. Anyone with a truly effective treatment would be trying very hard to get it licensed.

- *What are the motives and backgrounds of the suppliers?* If you can't find out, look elsewhere.

- *What does the official medical establishment think of the solution being offered, and why?* You may have to look far and wide for this answer, since a respected treatment in one part of the country might be viewed as fraud in another. The medical establishment is famous for rejecting solutions "not invented here" and is very conservative. Seek out all opinions and make your own decision.

- *Who can I talk to who's used this stuff, and how long have they used it?* The more the better, on both counts. If they can't put you in touch with users, try something else. Recognize that the results claimed for a treatment by only a few people or for a short period of time are virtually meaningless. People often get better for periods of time, with and without treatment. Ideally, listen to several people who have used a treatment for the longest possible period of time. Ask how they know they're doing better, what measures are they using, and how often they check. If something sounds too good to be true, it probably is.

Treatments supported by responsible, well-established AIDS information resources should have little trouble answering these questions. For those that can't, we must ask ourselves, *"Do I really want to be the first one on the block to try this?"* We must also avoid the temptation of joining the *"treatment of the month club"* which forms around new treatment options. Treatment must be separated from fad. Any effective treatment will usually take several weeks of use to demonstrate any significant benefits. People who bounce around from one treatment to the next are unlikely to achieve any benefits, and are even more unlikely to know what they are talking about.

Finally, pass on what you learn to others. Treatment information groups are anxious to collect feedback on the results people achieve.

CHALLENGE #3—FIGHTING BACK

AIDS ACTIVISM

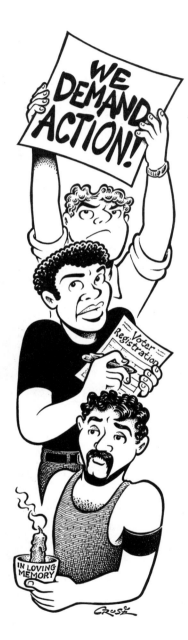

AIDS has stirred up a torrent of emotion in most of us. If we can sort out these feelings and have the clarity of mind to make the necessary medical decisions to stay alive, we are left with but one critical task in the war—fighting back. We must do both for ourselves—to overcome the feelings of rage and helplessness inside—and for our community. We owe it to ourselves, we owe it to every persecuted gay man and woman since the beginning of time, and especially, we owe it to every man, woman and child who has suffered at the hands of this cruel disease. Again, a point of view by the authors of this book: there is no excuse, no rationale which justifies not playing a direct role in fighting this war. It may be the single most important test of character and values any of us face in our lifetimes.

A sometimes callous and indifferent society will not break the back of this plague and medicine alone will not stop it. If there is a solution, it lies in the communal efforts of all those who care, all those who have been touched in any way by AIDS. Every angry activist has a role, every man who ever sat on a gay barstool has a role, and every regular Joe, auntie, cowboy, drag queen, jock, and leather stud has a role. The choice is simple:

find a way to get involved, to carry some of the weight on our shoulders, or participate in our own genocide.

Those most angry among us already shriek with frustration over the problems of this epidemic we haven't yet solved. Others acknowledge the burdens we have already carried while exhorting us on over the next hill.

Our own lives and the lives of all our friends are at stake, and our freedoms as well. Naturally, each of us must play our roles according to our individual gifts, capabilities, and temperaments. There are plenty of pathways to follow:

POLITICAL ACTIVISM:
Rage is a great source of energy. We can either let this energy tear us up internally or we can direct it at worthy targets. Ample outlets exist for channeling such energy, including direct political work, such as manning picket lines (for dozens of AIDS-related causes), writing to legislators, lobbying, challenging every homophobic bigot *every* time he or she speaks out, expressing your views in local elections, demanding a clear and sympathetic stand in return for your vote.

The message must be singular and clear to all who oppose us and take delight in our losses: *we are proud, gay, and enormously strong.*

Those who can't or won't work on the front lines can help support those who do. Financial contributions are needed by dozens of organizations, probably one in your own town, to carry on the work.

ECONOMIC ACTIVISM:
We needn't sit idly by while insurance companies, employers, landlords, or pharmaceutical companies exploit our suffering. When injustice exists, whether it be the insurance company which redlines the gay neighborhood or cuts services to an AIDS patient, an employer who fires people suspected of AIDS, or a drug company with a monopoly overcharges for treatment, *FIGHT BACK*! Small groups exist or can be organized quickly on an ad hoc basis to fight specific injustices. Sometimes, the law can be made to work on our behalf if we take the time and energy to do so. When the law won't help, pressure in the media and through public protest can often quickly right a wrong. The business interests and public images of our exploiters are usually vulnerable enough to permit quick solutions for those willing to resist.

COMMUNITY SERVICE:
The gay community has established a standard for the world in caring for our sick. Volunteers are needed in every major city for a variety of roles: tending directly for the sick, "buddy" programs, meals-on-wheels services, office help in AIDS organizations, hot-line work, fund-raising, educational efforts (including writing and advertising). Such involvement redirects rage into productive work and directly relieves feelings of helplessness.

Again, if you can't or won't do the work, send money to support those who will.

COUNSELING SERVICE:
If you've "gotten it together" yourself, join an organization and help others reach a similar state; not all have found it so easy. Groups like Shanti Project train and make good use of one-on-one counselors to help others through times of crisis. If you're a professional with special skills, it's time to share them with your community.

EDUCATIONAL SERVICE:
Many of the societal problems associated with AIDS result from misinformation or a lack of information. Taking responsibility for helping educate others can result in a smoother ride for the community as whole. For those with the skills, put the time in on community service projects to educate our fellow citizens. Educate politicians with correspondence. When raving bigots spout misinformation on call-in talk shows, call in yourself and set the record straight. Those who have either the skill and the opportunity to educate through the

media, must do so without hesitation or concern for personal backlash. In our daily lives, politely challenge every bit of misinformation or cruelty directed against people with AIDS, every notion of casual contagion, every warped view which blames the victims. If this means coming out at work, with friends, or family, maybe it's about time. The most widespread crime of the Holocaust of World War II was the silence of those who knew but didn't speak up.

EVERYDAY LIVING:
Find a way to devote at least some portion of your time, every week or month, to an AIDS-related cause. It might mean spending a little more time than usual with friends who are sick, or staying in closer touch with a friend who is ill in another city. If you have friends who are ill, ask yourself,

Have I asked him what he need or wants from me?

Am I am doing all I can, all my friend(s) wants me to do?

Can I help more with my time, my money, my skills?

Am I avoiding the subject, for my own comfort, to the detriment of others?

Just what have I done this day, this week, this month, to help?

A FINAL WORD

The one thing we know for sure won't help—about our own feelings of rage and helplessness, or the community's profound needs in time of crisis—is doing nothing. If we passively accept an unfair fate for ourselves, our friends, or our community, if we overlook the options available to us, and simply "wait and see" if a solution will come our way, our prophecy of helplessness becomes our inevitable fate.

It is inconceivable that we will again face another crisis of such dimensions in our lifetime. This may be our generation's greatest opportunity to demonstrate—to ourselves, our community, and the world around us— the strength, love, and courage of being free and liberated gay men. We can and will conquer this plague, stand tall for our brothers in need, and shatter the closet door forever. There is, and should be, no looking back.

RESOURCES—Appendix

RESOURCES—APPENDIX

The amount and type of information available about AIDS is stagger-ing—books, newsletters, hotlines, videos, support services, political and legal services, research findings. One can make a full time job of exploring it all. One of the great strengths of our community in this crisis is that we have developed our own information distribution channels to supplement more traditional resources. The depth and quality of resources which have been assembled, to a large extent by the community, give testimony to the ways which we have learned to help ourselves and our own. History records no other group that has organized and supported itself in time of crisis quite the way this community has.

We can't assume that any single expert will have accurate answers to all our questions. Keeping up with AIDS information is difficult even for people who work in the field full time. Taking responsibility by learning to use information tools effectively enables us to learn inde-pendently and gain confidence in our ability to chart a course through the seeming maze of facts, speculation, and possible misinformation.

In making use of available resources, it helps to begin by sorting out our own information needs, deciding what we really need to know. Some people express AIDS anxiety by compulsively seeking all pos-sible information about AIDS. In doing so, they often lose all sense of their priorities and get bogged down in trivial detail. We don't need to know everything, digest every bit of data, to set our own course or action. When we take time to think through our informa-tion needs before picking up the phone, the time and energy we spend working with the resources is used more efficiently. It also al-lows the service organizations to make better use of their time. Noth-ing is more frustrating than a constantly busy phone number.

The following appendix provides but a brief overview of what is out there. For every organization listed, there are perhaps ten more un-listed. No slight is intended for groups or services whose names do not appear here—only a shortness of pages and a limit to our knowl-edge. Resources are listed in two broad categories—*COMMUNITY SERVICES* and *SUPPORT MATERIALS* (reading and videos).

COMMUNITY SERVICES:

- General information resources and hotlines
- Treatment information and hotlines
- Legal services
- Political action
- Computerized information networks

Where information on local resources is lacking, the national network numbers, listed can provide referrals. Local numbers, while limited, can give you a starting place for learning in your region. Some numbers are provided for those cities known to have large gay populations afflicted by AIDS.

SUPPORT MATERIALS:

This is a listing of supplemental materials—books, articles, and video-tapes—which expand on the subjects addressed in individual chapters of this book.

Community Services

General information resources and hotlines (national, local, and international).

There are at least several hundred AIDS organizations and social service agencies, so we cannot list them all here. There is probably an AIDS hotline that covers your geographical area. That hotline will have a directory of local organizations. To get a local hotline number, not listed here, look in the phone book or call your information operator and ask. If you can't find one that way, call one of the national toll-free hotlines and ask for a local or regional referral.

NATIONAL:

National AIDS Hotline (Centers for Disease Control), (referrals to local resources).　　800-342-AIDS

National AIDS Network, (non-government)　　202-546-2424
729 8th St. SE, Washington, DC 20003
(referrals to local resources)

LOCAL:

ATLANTA　　404-872-0600
AID Atlanta, 811 Cyprus Street NW, Atlanta,
GA 30308

BOSTON　　800-235-2331
AIDS Action Committee, 661 Boylston St.　　(Mass. only)
Suite 4, Boston, MA 02116

CHICAGO　　312-871-5777
*Howard Brown Memorial Clinic AIDS
Action Project*, 2676 N. Halsted, Chicago, IL
60614

DENVER　　303-837-0166
Colorado AIDS Project, P.O. Box 18529,
Denver, CO 80218

HOUSTON　　713-524-2437
KS AIDS Foundation, 3317 Montrose, Box
1155, Houston, TX 77006

LOS ANGELES　　213-876-8951
AIDS Project Los Angeles, 7362 Santa
Monica Blvd. Los Angeles, CA 90046

NEW YORK   212-807-6664
Gay Men's Health Crisis, Inc. 132 W. 24th,
New York, NY 10011

People with AIDS Coalition, Inc. 263A   212-627-1810
W. 19th St, Room 125, New York, NY 10011

SAN FRANCISCO   415-864-4376
San Francisco AIDS Foundation Hotline,
333 Valencia, 4th Floor San Francisco, CA
94103

Shanti Project, 525 Howard, San Francisco   415-777-2273
CA 94105

AIDS Interfaith Network, 890 Hayes, San   415-558-9644.
Francisco, CA 94117

INTERNATIONAL:

CANADA   403-426-1516
AIDS Network of Edmunton, 11303 102nd
Ave., Edmunton, Alberta, T5K 0P6

AIDS Committee of Toronto, c/o Hassle
Free Clinic, 556 Church St., 2nd Floor,
Toronto, Ontario, M4Y 2E3

Comite SIDA du Quebec, 3757 rue
Prud'homme, Montreal, Quebec, H4A 3H8

ENGLAND
Capitol Gay, 38 Mt. Pleasant, London MC1X
OAP

FRANCE
Association des Gais Medecins, 45 rue
Sedaind, 75011 Paris.

NETHERLANDS
AIDS Policy Coordinator, Jan K. van
Wijngaarden, M.D., Buro G.V.O. Prins
Henderiklaand 12, 1075 BB Amsterdam

PUERTO RICO
Latin American STD Center, Rio Piedras,   809-754-8118
Centro Medico, 00922

- TREATMENT INFORMATION AND RESOURCES

AMFAR (American Foundation for AIDS Research), 40 W. 57th St., Suite 406, New York, NY 10019 (directory of clinical drug trials on a subscription basis)	212-333-3118
Dcoumentation of Aids Issues and Research Foundation (archive of AIDS-related publications, research articles, and media stories), 25 Taylor St. Suite 616, San Francisco, CA 94102.	415-928-0292
Gay Men's Health Crisis, Inc., 132 W. 24th, New York, NY 10011, Attn: Dr. Barry Gingell	212-807-6664
Project Inform, 25 Taylor St. Suite 618, San Francisco CA 94102 (hotline/ information on available experimental treatments)	(Nat) 1-800-822-7222 (CA) 1- 800-334-7422 415-928-0293
Healing Alternatives Buyers Club, P.O. Box 411107, San Francisco, CA 94141 (information and access to treatments)	415-621-4346
Guerrilla Clinics referrals (information and access to treatments)	415-647-8561
PWA Health Group, Box 234 70-A Greenwich Ave, NY, NY 10011 (information and access to treatments)	212-995-5846

- LEGAL SERVICES (additional legal services are often available through local AIDS organizations)

Lambda Legal Defense League, 666 Broadway, New York, NY 10012	212-995-8585
National Gay Rights Advocates, 8389 Santa Monica Blvd., Suite 202, Los Angeles, CA 90069	213-650-6200

- POLITICAL ACTION

Gay Rights National Lobby/AIDS Project, PO Box 1892, Washington, DC 20012.	202-546-1801.
Mobilization Against Aids, San Francisco CA	415-431-4660
National Gay and Lesbian Task Force, 80 Fifth Avenue, New York, NY 10011.	1-800-221-7044 (3 to 9 PM, EST)

- COMPUTERIZED INFORMATION NETWORKS

CAIN, the Computerized AIDS Information Network, is an AIDS-specific service available on the Delphi information utility. CAIN has up-to-the-minute information on many AIDS topics, including a monthly review of AIDS medical literature (abstracts of about 250 new articles each month). For details on CAIN, contact the Gay and Lesbian Community Services Center, 1213 N. Highland Avenue, Hollywood, CA 90038. (213) 464-7400, extension 277.

Connect through:

DELPHI information service, 3 Blackstone Street, Cambridge, MA 02139	1-800-554-4005

MEDLINE, a system provided by the National Library of Medicine, gives online access to a database of about 5 million literature citations and abstracts (not the full text of the documents) published since 1966. MEDLINE covers approximately 3,400 journals and is updated monthly, following all aspects of biomedicine, including allied health fields such as nursing and drug reactions, as well as social science topics related to health care.

For detailed performance and costs, see: *"Computer searching of the medical literature:* an evaluation of MEDLINE searching systems," Haynes RB et al., Ann Intern Med, Nov. 1985; 103(5):812-6.

Paperchase is a very easy-to-use, menu-driven method for accessing the MEDLINE database. Developed by Beth Israel Hospital, Boston, Paperchase is available on CompuServe, described elsewhere. It covers all the material in MEDLINE dating back to 1975—over 3,000,000 references from some 3,400 journals. The average charge per search is $7 to $8. Although the actual document cannot be retrieved online, you can order a copy electronically at a cost of $6 per article. Access through either:

CompuServe, 5000 Arlington Centre Blvd.,   614-457-8600
PO Box 20212, Columbus, OH 43220,

Dialog Information Services, 3460 Hillview   1-800-227-1927
Avenue, Palo Alto, CA 94304

Another excellent computerized resource is the *Medical Data Exchange*. For information on access, call the number listed below.

Medical Data Exchange, On-Line AIDS   1-800-633-3667
Update Service.

Support Materials

READINGS:

CHAPTER 1 — Health in the Age of AIDS

AIDS: A Self-Care Manual, editors Betty Clare Moffatt, Judith Speigel, Steve Parrish, Michael Helquest. AIDS Project Los Angeles, 1987.

Illness as a Metaphor, Susan Sontag. Farrar, Straus, and Giroux, New York, 1977.

Loving Someone Gay, Don Clark. Celestial Arts, Millbrae, 1977, 1979.

Positively Gay, Betty Berzon and Robert Leighton. Celestial Arts, Millbrae, 1972.

Society and the Healthy Homosexual, George Weinberg. St. Martin's Press.

The Homosexual Matrix, C.A. Tripp. Signet, New York, 1975, 1977.

The Turning Point: Science, Society, and the Rising Culture, Fritjof Capra. Bantam, Toronto, 1982.

When Bad Things Happen to Good People, H. S. Kushner. Avon Books, New York, 1981.

CHAPTER 2 — Sexual Practices

Men Loving Men: Images of Male Sexuality, Jack Morin. Down There Press, Burlingame, 1980.

Men Loving Men: A Gay Sex Guide & Consciousness Book, Mitch Walker. Gay Sunshine Press, San Francisco, 1977.

The Complete Guide to Safe Sex, The Institute for Advanced Study of Human Sexuality. Specific Press, San Francisco, 1987.

The Hot'n Healthy Times, (a newspaper devoted to safe sex), San Francisco AIDS Foundation, 333 Valencia, 4th floor, San Francisco, CA 94103.

The Condom Book: The Essential for Men and Women, Jane Everett and Walter Glanz. Nal/Signet, 1987.

Terrific Sex in Fearful Times, Brooks Peters. St. Martin's Press, New York, due 1988.

A Manual for Safe Sex: Intimacy Without Fear, Donald Kilby. Publisher's Marketing Service, Los Angeles, 1987.

Safe Sex, Harvey Fierstein. Atheneum, 1987.

Facing It: A Novel of AIDS, Paul Reed. Gay Sunshine Press, San Francisco, 1984.

Safestud, Max Exander. Male.

Lovesex, Max Exander. Male.

CHAPTER 3 — The Role of Stress

A Gradual Awakening, Stephen Levine. Anchor, Garden City, 1979.

Guide to Stress Reduction, L. John Mason. Peace Press, Culver City, 1980.

Journey of Awakening: A Meditator's Guidebook, Ram Dass. Bantam, New York, 1978.

Mind as a Healer, Mind as a Slayer: A Holistic Approach to Preventing Stress Disorders, Kenneth Pelletier. Delta Books, New York, 1977.

Stress Without Distress, Hans Selye. Lippincott, New York, 1974.

The Massage Book, George Downing. Random House, New York, 1972.

The Psychology of Consciousness, Robert Ornstein. W. H. Freeman, San Francisco, 1972.

The Relaxation Response, Herbert Benson. Avon, New York, 1975.

The Stress of Life, Hans Selye. McGraw-Hill, New York, 1956.

CHAPTER 4 — Substance Use and Abuse

A Step Over the Line: a No Nonsense Guide to Recognize and Treat Cocaine Dependency. Harper & Row, San Francisco, 1980.

Adult Children of Alcoholics, Jane Geringer Woitistz. Health Communication Inc. Harper & Row, San Francisco, 1983.

Al Anon, Third Edition, Alcoholics Anonymous World Services, Inc., New York, 1976.

I'll Quit Tomorrow, Vernon Johnson. Harper & Row, San Francisco, 1980.

It Will Never Happen to Me, Claudia Black. M.A.C., Denver, 1982.

The Twelve Steps of Alcoholics Anonymous, Interpreted by the Hazelton Foundation. Harper & Row, New York, 1974.

CHAPTER 5 — Social Support

A Family Matter: A Parent's Guide to Homosexuality, Charles Silverstein. McGraw-Hill, New York, 1977.

Beyond Acceptance: Parents of Lesbians and Gays Talk about their Experiences, Carolyn W. Griffith, Marian & Arthur Wirth. Prentice-Hall, Englewood, New Jersey, 1986.

Epidemic of Courage: Facing AIDS in America, Lon Nunsgesser. St. Martin's Press, New York, 1986.

Man to Man: Gay Couples in America, Charles Silverstein. William Morrow, New York, 1981.

The Art of Loving, Erich Fromm. Harper & Row, New York, 1956.

The Male Couple: How Relationships Develop, David McWhirter and Andrew Mattison. Prentice-Hall, 1984.

The Screaming Room, Barbara Peabody. Oaktree, San Diego, 1986.

When A Friend Has AIDS, San Francisco AIDS Foundation, 333 Valencia Street, 4th Floor, San Francisco, CA 94103, (415) 864-4376.

CHAPTER 6 — Exercise and Nutrition

Stretching, Bob Anderson. Shelter Publications, Bolinas, 1980.

Swimming for Total Fitness: a Progressive Aerobic Program, Jane Katz and Nancy Bruning. Doubleday, New York, 1981.

The New Aerobics, Kenneth Cooper. Bantam, Toronto, 1970.

The Pilates Method of Physical and Mental Conditioning, Philip Friedman and Gail Eisen. Doubleday, Garden City, 1980.

Diet for a Happy Heart, Jeanne Jones. 101 Productions, San Francisco, 1975.

Diet for a Small Planet, Frances Lappe. Ballantine, New York, 1971.

Eat Right, Eat Well, the Italian Way, Edward Giobbi and Richard Wolff. Knopf, New York, 1985.

The Pritikin Promise, Nathan Pritikin. Pocket, New York, 1983.

CHAPTER 7 — Fighting for Our Lives

AIDS: Facts and Issues, Victor Gong and Norman Rednick, editors. Rutgers, New Brunswick, 1986.

Anatomy of an Illness, Norman Cousins. Bantam Books, Toronto, 1982.

Christianity, Social Tolerance, and Homosexuality, John Boswell. University of Chicago Press, Chicago, 1980.

Death, the Final Stage of Growth, Elizabeth Kubler-Ross. Prentice-Hall, Englewood Cliffs, 1975.

Focus: A Review of AIDS Research (a monthly review of information relevant to health care and service providers). AIDS Health Project, 333 Valencia Street, 4th floor, San Francisco, CA 94103.

Getting Well Again, Carl O. Simonton, Stephanie Matthews-Simonton, and James L. Creighton. Bantam Books, New New York, 1978.

Healing from Within: Psychological Techniques to Help the Mind and the Body, Dennis Jaffe. Fireside, New York, 1980.

Homosexuality, A History, Vern L. Bullough. Meridian, New American Library, New York, 1979.

I Thought People Like That Killed Themselves: Lesbian and Gay Suicide, Eric Rolfes. Grey Fox Press, San Francisco, 1983.

Love, Medicine, and Miracles: Lessons Learned about Self-Healing from a Surgeon's Experience with Exceptional Patients, Bernie Siegal. Harper & Row, 1986.

Man's Search for Meaning, Victor Frankl. Pocket Books, New York, 1963.

Mobilizing Against AIDS: The Unfinished Story of a Virus, The Institute of Medicine of the National Academy of Sciences. Harvard University, Cambridge, 1986.

No Magic Bullet: A Social History of Venereal Disease in the United States since 1880 (with a new chapter on AIDS), Allan Brandt. Oxford University Press, Oxford, 1987.

Notes On Living Until We Say Goodbye: A Personal Guide, Lon G. Nunsgesser. St. Martin's Press, due 1988.

Questions and Answers on Death and Dying, Elizabeth Kubler-Ross. MacMillan, New York, 1974.

Sex and Germs: The Politics of AIDS, Cindy Patton. South End, Boston, 1985.

Surviving and Thriving with AIDS: Hints for the Newly Diagnosed, edited by Michael Callen. People with AIDS Coalition. Available from National AIDS Network.

The Church and the Homosexual, John McNeill. Sheed, Andrews, and McMeel, Inc., 1976.

The Courage to Grieve: Creative Living, Recovery, and Growth Through Grief, Judy Tatelbaum. Harper & Row, New York, 1980.

The Meaning of Anxiety, Rollo May. Washington Square Press, New York, 1950.

VIDEOTAPES

Volunteer Training, Shanti Project. Shanti, a widely-respected patient care organization, has made its complete volunteer training program available on videotape. The tapes can be used by any group wishing to start an organization to provide volunteer counseling to people with AIDS, their loved ones and friends. These training materials are designed to be used both as a resource by the organizers of a new group and in the training of volunteer counselors. The Shanti Project, 860 Hayes Street, San Francisco, CA 94117, 415-558-9644.

AIDS: Care Beyond The Hospital, is a videotape training program designed as a teaching tool for health care providers who are, or will wbe, working with people with AIDS in the home. This material is not designed for lay people or general audiences, but would be of value to organizations seeking to build a home health care program. For details contact the San Francisco AIDS Foundation, 333 Valencia Street, Fourth Floor, San Francisco, CA 94103, 415-864-4376.

AIDS: Putting the Puzzle Together is a series of videotapes designed for the health care community. The tapes share the experience of professional care providers serving people with AIDS. Inservice Video Productions, 1191 Carey Drive, Concord, CA 94520, 415-827-2711. SAFE SEX GUIDES.

Hot Living: Erotic Stories About Safer Sex, is a collection of sixteen sizzling stories that will stoke your fire and give you some good ideas to try out in real life. Royalties are donated to the Gay Men's Health Crisis, a New York City organization. Alyson Publications, Dept. P-6, 40 Plympton Street, Boston, MA 02118, $8 plus $1 shipping.

Lifeguard, The Safe Sex Video, shows it all—in living color! Prominent sex stars demonstrate fabulous techniques you can use. It may be playing at a video store near you; if not, order from HIS Video, 9333 Oso Avenue, Chatsworth, CA 91311, 1-800-458-4336, $39.95.

Relaxation and Healing and Season for Health cover relaxation and imagery as applied to cancer therapy. Learning for Health, 1314 Westwood Boulevard, #107, Los Angeles, CA 90024.

Conditioned Relaxation, for Progressive relaxation. Center for Integral Medicine, PO Box 967, Pacific Palisades, CA 90272.

Stress Reduction First Aid Tape, including relaxation and sleep induction. Halpern Sounds, 620 Taylor Way, #14, Belmont, CA 94002.

Exploring the Heart of Healing, with Stephen Levine and Ram Dass. San Francisco AIDS Foundation, 333 Valencia, 4th floor, San Francisco, CA 94103.

AUDIO TAPES

Relaxation and Visualization, William Vitiello. The UCSF AIDS Health Project, UCSF Box 0884, San Francisco, CA 94143-0884.

Meditation: An Instructional Cassette, Daniel Goleman. Psychology Today Cassettes, P.O. Box 278, Pratt Station, Brooklyn, NY 11205.

Meditation of the Heart: A Guided Visualization, Ram Dass. Psychology Today Cassettes, P.O. Box 278, Pratt Station, Brooklyn, NY 11205.

INDEX—Strategies for Survival

316

Production Notes

This book was produced by and for the gay community. To keep the selling cost of the book as low as possible, desktop publishing technologies were used instead of traditional typesetting methods.

Text was written and formatted on an IBM™ AT using Microsoft™ Word. Publication masters were printed on a Quadram™ Quadlaser laser printer using fonts by Bitstream™.

Proofing was done by hand, both at St. Martin's Press in New York and in the gay communities of Sausalito and San Francisco, California.

ABOUT THE AUTHORS

Martin Delaney is an AIDS activist, independent businessman, and co-founder of Project Inform, a well-known AIDS treatment information resource and originator of the community research movement. He is often featured in the media (ABC Nightline, Donahue, 20-20, WSJ, etc.) discussing AIDS issues and speaking out as a critic of government AIDS policy. His work includes personal contact with hundreds of AIDS/ARC patients, meetings with the U.S. FDA and National Institutes of Health, and input to major gay organizations. He is the author of widely-quoted treatment information and has done work for the National Institute on Drug Abuse. As a businessman and a writer, he provides educational design, negotiating, and media services to major corporations, is in demand as a seminar presenter/lecturer, and writes and produces seminars and educational videos on collaborative negotiation, equal opportunity, consultative selling, and quality assurance.

Peter Goldblum is a pioneer in the study of gay psychology. For the past fifteen years he has been actively involved in clinical practice, program administration, lecturing, teaching and writing on topics related to gay health and psychology. He has contributed articles and book chapters to both professional and lay publications, including article on AIDS and Suicide, HIV antibody testing, counseling, health planning, and the development of support services for health professionals working with AIDS. He served as the first deputy director of the AIDS Health Project, at the University of California, San Francisco, where he headed the prevention services and supervised the AIDS and Substance Abuse Program. He currently serves as a member of the AIDS Task Force at the Pacific Graduate School of Psychology, Menlo Park and practices clinical psychology in San Francisco.

Joe Brewer is a psychotherapist in private practice and an activist for gay causes. He is the other co-founder of Project Inform and a former executive director of the widely-respected Pacific Center. He served in the development of the AIDS Health Project of the University of California at San Francisco and has been a seminal voice in the foundation of several other agencies and services. Before AIDS, he was instrumental, along with Peter Goldblum, in the development of the "B group," a noted pioneering health support service for chronic hepatitis patients which is the direct ancestor of the processes and thinking which have come to fruition in this book. Joe, who is strongly tied into the national AIDS network, currently manages a thriving clinical psychology practice with a heavy emphasis on AIDS issues, and, along with Martin Delaney, is often seen conducting standing-room-only town meetings in San Francisco under the banner of Project Inform.